THE NEW MEDICAL FOLLIES

THE
NEW MEDICAL FOLLIES

An Encyclopedia of Cultism and Quackery in These United States, with Essays on The Cult of Beauty, The Craze for Reduction, Rejuvenation, Eclecticism, Bread and Dietary Fads, Physical Therapy, and a Forecast as to the Physician of the Future.

By

MORRIS FISHBEIN, M.D.

EDITOR OF THE JOURNAL OF THE AMERICAN MEDICAL ASSOCIATION
AND OF HYGEIA, THE HEALTH MAGAZINE

NEW YORK

BONI AND LIVERIGHT
1927

PREFACE

The essays here presented have appeared in such periodicals as the *American Mercury*, the *Haldeman-Julius Monthly*, the *Journal of the American Medical Association*, *Hygeia*, *the Health Magazine*, *The Nation's Business*, the *Delineator*, and in the newspapers. All have been revised and amended for this volume. A few chapters appear here for the first time.

MORRIS FISHBEIN.

CONTENTS

THE NEW MEDICAL FOLLIES

THE NEW
MEDICAL FOLLIES

CHAPTER I

AN ENCYCLOPEDIA OF CULTS AND QUACKERIES

OF all the nations of the world, the United States is most afflicted by its healers. Besides those holding the degree M.D., signifying doctor of medicine and, nowadays, some seven years of study following high school graduation, a host of queer practitioners pervade the medical field. They have conferred on themselves strange combinations of letters, indicating the peculiar systems of healing which a somewhat lax system of legislation and law enforcement permits them to practice on an unwary public. One of the marks of the charlatan is the use in advertising of such an alphabetic appendage.

Cult follows cult and quackery succeeds quackery, frequently with amazing rapidity. Moreover, many cults seem to be definitely confined to small districts and fail to come to light in the available literature on the subject, or even in a careful investigation. Then, too, a single temporarily successful cult like chiropractic—itself the child of osteopathy and magnetic healing—gives birth to many offshoots which again propagate more bizarre offspring and unusual hybrids. A complete picture of the far cical scene would require endless research. The United States unquestionably bears the palm in every class so far as healing cults are concerned.

A cult is "excessive devotion to some person, idea, or thing, especially when pursued as an intellectual fad by a body of enthusiastic, self-constituted admirers." As applied particularly to medicine, a "sectarian" is one who in his practice follows a dogma, tenet, or principle, based on the authority of its promulgator to the exclusion of demonstration and experience. As is at once apparent, it must have a leader. These are usually men of powerful personality, intensely egocentric, frequently young and handsome, but often merely shrewd with the shrewdness of long experience and old age. Sometimes they are self-deluded, but more often they are consciously deluding. Likely as not they feel themselves and announce themselves as divinely inspired. The combination of priesthood and the healing art is as old as mankind itself. James Huneker asked: "What is the difference between a false and a true prophet? Aren't they both fakirs?" The lives of the cultist leaders inspire in any careful analyst the belief that few of them suffer from inordinate honesty of either conviction or practice.

The scientific medicine of to-day is based on the discoveries made in the fundamental sciences. It holds to no single theory as to the causation of disease and it does not insist correspondingly that the successful treatment of disease depends on the use of any single method of manipulation or administration. The cults may be classified easily into mental healing cults, mechanical cults, electric cults, nature cults and similar divisions, since they adhere definitely to such single devices. Other cults may be classed merely as non-medical, since they deprecate the use of medicaments. They are founded, moreover, on peculiar fallacies with relation to the anatomy of the body, on misconceptions of certain physiologic functions, or on exaggerations of the relative importance of certain parts of the body in maintaining it in a constant state of health; these cults avoid the fundamental sciences as far as possible. Rather than attempt to correlate the fallacies on which the cults are based with established knowledge, cultist leaders are inclined to deny flatly the facts that have been demonstrated. Of germs and their causation of disease, they take little cognizance, referring constantly to the "germ theory." Many cultist leaders denounce the eating of meat because of some weird notions of body chemistry. Others employ apparatus of such intricacies as would bring a flush of envy to the cheek of Rube Goldberg; mechanically such machinery excites the ridicule of the humblest tyro in the science of physics. The complacency with which cultist leaders dispose of the fundamental facts of science in promoting their views may be taken as sound evidence of their essential eccentricities.

'A

Aerotherapy. Among the hundred or more types of healing offered to the sophisticated is aerotherapy. Obviously aerotherapy means treatment by air, but in this instance hot air is particularly concerned. The patient is baked in a hot oven. Heat relieves pain and produces an increased flow of blood to the part heated. The blood aids in removing waste products and brings to the part the substances that overcome infection. There is nothing essentially wrong about hot air therapy.

Since the time of Hippocrates and indeed even in Biblical legend men have availed themselves of the healing powers existing in nature. The light and heat of the sun, the burning steam from natural hot springs, the dry air of the desert, and even the buffeting of the waves of the sea have been used for physical stimulation in overcoming disease. It has remained for the astute commercial minds of our progressive land to incorporate these qualities for their personal gain.

Aerotherapy as one department of physical therapy becomes a cult when it is used to the exclusion of all other forms of healing. In New York a progressive quack established an institute equipped with special devices for pouring hot air over various portions of the body. He issued a beautiful brochure, illustrated with the likenesses of beautiful damsels in various states of négligée, smiling the smile of the satisfied, under his salubrious ministrations. In this document appeared incidentally the claim that hot air will cure anything from ague to zoster. The same claim has been made by the faith healers and the apostles of manipulation. But the first call it Christian Science and the second call it chiropractic.

Alereos System. Here is a system of drugless healing which "recognized the human body as a wonderful and perfect machine, which, properly adjusted and taken care of, will run without friction." It emanates from Brooklyn. "The Alereos system," says the folder, "in relation to the human machine, occupies the place of the skilled mechanic to the disabled engine. It searches for the causes of the trouble and seeks to remove them by its tools. These are the hands, aided by several mechanical appliances and vibrations." The home office supplies heat and mechanical vibration with "several specially constructed apparati (sic)." Not content to sell its simple hot air and vibration treatments on their merits, the Alereos system plays strongly on the osteopathic and chiropractic claims of contractions and pinched nerves, and condemns all drug treatment as poisoning. It is the acme of exploitation of the sweat bath and massage. One takes ten treatments for twenty-five dollars *in advance;* obviously, the cost is little, provided one is not fooled into neglecting tuberculosis or ulcer of the stomach, which are among the conditions mentioned in the Alereos folder.

Astral Healing.   Casanova, international lover and charlatan, tells at great length of his delving into magic, of the drawing of horoscopes and of astrology.   The mystery of the stars has always had fascination for the multitude and it would have been strange, indeed, if some astute healer had failed to take advantage of this folly in the founding of a cult. The Astral healers advertise in foreign language newspapers.   They read the diagnosis from the horoscope and then make an additional charge for giving the advice indicated by their readings.

Autohemic Therapy.   For many years one L. D. Rogers was the head and chief owner of the National Medical University of Chicago.   The school was a low-grade institution, virtually a diploma mill. Rogers is a promoter of medical schemes and fancies.   Like many other cultist leaders he is constantly founding societies of which he is the chief panjandrum.   Once he was the permanent secretary of the National Association of Panpathic Physicians, apparently an attempt to organize all the comical cultists into a single group.   However, the society had only a brief existence and the permanent secretary was quite temporary.   Then he began to exploit a cancer serum and he organized the American

Cancer Research Society, L. D. Rogers, president. Finally, he got the notion called "autohemic therapy." "It consists," he says, "in giving the patient a solution made by attenuating, hemolizing, incubating and potentizing a few drops of his or her own blood, and administering it according to a refined technic developed by the author." Playing the game to the limit, Rogers also advertises a one-hundred-dollar mail order course for other physicians. He wrote a book called "Autohemic Therapy" and organized the Autohemic Practitioners. Newspaper publicity in the form of full-page advertisements and clever press agentry fetch the come-ons for the course. The appeal is made cleverly to the anti-medical cultists of all varieties by the slogan "without use of bugs or drugs." A clever and shrewd old fakir is L. D. Rogers! There is not an iota of scientific evidence that his method or his system ever cured anybody of anything.

Autology. E. R. Moras, M.D., founder of Autology, finally arrived in the "booby-hatch." Before that, however, he had achieved a considerable following through advertising in the press, and through exploitation along the lines established by Elbert Hubbard. Indeed, Elbert said of Autology: "Dr. Moras has written a Commonsense Book on Autology, and by so doing, placed the Standard of the Creed of Health farther to the front than any man who has lived for a thousand years." Ah well,

Elbert was never much given to conservative statements! As might be expected Moras also had the support of *Physical Culture,* Bernarr Macfadden's major opus; of J. H. Tilden of Denver, who has some fads of his own, and even of Luther Burbank.

Autology is a system of stereotyped hygienic and dietetic advice sandwiched in between a lot of pseudo-science and bad counsel. It is essentially another preachment of Ecclesiastes' urge for moderation in all things. Unfortunately it was carried to the point at which Elbert Hubbard said, "Moderation, equality, work and love—you need no other physician." Moras exploited his book at anywhere from $10 to $2, and on the side sold some patent medicines. Finally, his eccentricity went beyond the bounds of legal sufferance. He was arrested for insulting a woman on a train; he attempted to blackmail Leon Mandel out of a million dollars, and appealed to the President of the United States to help him collect $50,000 from Parke-Davis and Company. So his friends put him in a sanatorium!

Auto-Science. An Auto-Science Institute is conducted in San Francisco, devoted, it appears, to practical psychology, scientific serums and suggestive therapeutics. The watchword is "Law of Creative Energy." Regular lessons can be had for four weeks on trial, but the diploma, the degree and the "Auto-Science" text-book cost $35, which is a special reduction from the sum of $50, the regular fee for the course. The high priest, Dr. E. C. Feyrer, presents testimonials of grateful imbeciles who have been cured of all sorts of things. It appears that not only can you heal yourself, but you can help others by mental broadcasting. Is there no protection against this sort of thing? Must one be healed even when he enjoys ill-health?

Autotherapy. This pleasant little idea grew in the mind of a homeopath, presumably obsessed with the homeopathic slogan "similia similibus curantur," or "like cures like." Dr. Charles H. Duncan of New York was able to have his views promulgated through some of the good medical journals and their strangeness secured him unusually great newspaper recognition. "Autotherapy," as the name implies, is "self-therapy" or "natural therapy." The word "nature" is a term to conjure with in cultism. Carrying the idea of the "hair of the dog that bit you" to its ultimate interpretation, Duncan recommends the healing of boils by cooking up and swallowing the matter from the boil; for dysentery he filters the excretions and injects the fluid that filters through; for tuberculosis he filters the sputum and injects the filtrate. He claims all sorts of cures. It is the belief of competent authorities that the system has no basis in scientific knowledge and that the results secured, if any, are merely such as follow injections of foreign substances of any kind into the body.

B

Bio-Dynamo-Chromatic-Diagnosis and Therapy.
Whenever the irregulars in the healing art assemble
for the purpose of exchanging trade secrets and telling each other how good they are, George Starr
White, M.D., F.S.Sc. (Lond.), D.C., Ph.D., LL.D.,
Los Angeles, is among those present. He was "second vice-president" of the Allied Medical Associations in 1918. He is also opposed to vaccination and
helps out the American Medical Liberty League.
White was graduated from the New York Homeopathic Medical College when he was forty-two years
old. He played with Abrams' spondylotherapy (see
later) and also pushed Fitzgerald's "zone therapy"
(see later). Then he developed the fancy-name system that combines a lot of hocus-pocus—it seems one
diagnoses disease by a "Sympathetic Vagal Reflex."
To elicit the said phenomenon, the patient faces
east or west and his abdomen is thumped until a dull
area is found. Then colored lights are thrown on
the abdomen and the thumping is continued. A ruby
and blue light with associated dullness means one
thing and a green light combination another. That
is to say, Dr. White says so; really, it doesn't mean
anything. Once Dr. White took a flier in the patent
medicine business. The F.S.Sc. (Lond.), with
which he is endowed, means "Fellow of the Incorporated Society of Science, Letters and Arts of

London, Ltd." Lots of people who play the same game as White have the same letters. The cost of the elegant diploma is about $5. Sometimes White also puts after his name D.C., Ph.D., LL.D. No one knows where he got those. The method was given a beautiful send-off in Mr. Macfadden's *Physical Culture* magazine by Dr. Edwin F. Bowers in February, 1918. Dr. Bowers is not a doctor of medicine and the only M.D. he has is the one Macfadden gives him. Strange how the same names recur again and again in these stories of the ghoul-like activities of the harpies who live by exploiting the sick!

In 1925, White produced the last word in this fancy business, the Rithmo-Chrome and Duo-Colors. He has a lot of books to sell and a lot of apparatus. For instance, in his latest announcement, Figure 10 shows a "person sitting on a Filteray Cushion and receiving Filtered Ultrared Rays while doing Rithmo-Chrome breathing and inhaling Oxygen-Vapor or Medicated Vapor and at the time getting therapeutic effect of the magnetic forces of the earth, as he is grounded and facing exactly north and south." If the Duo-Colors are added to this, Dr. White affirms, the patient is certainly getting "Natural Methods Condenst." And if he isn't getting that, what is he getting?

Biological Blood-Washing. This utter humbug is accredited to Benedict Lust, of whom more later.

He is one of the king pins of the naturopathy cult.
Under "naturopathy" his record will be made apparent.

C

Chiropractic. This apotheosis of the backbone
first saw the light in Davenport, Iowa, in 1894.
D. D. Palmer, founder of the cult, was a magnetic healer who had sojourned briefly in Kirksville,
Mo., under the tutelage of Andrew Still, founder of
osteopathy. An experiment on a deaf janitor convinced him that all disease is the result of displaced
bones in the spine, pressing on the nerves that pass
from the spinal cord. This being the case, disease is
cured by pushing the bones back. No one as yet has
explained what makes them stay back. Since the propounding of this system, scientists have spent many
hours of research on the question, but have found
that the very basis of the cult is a fallacy. Actually
the pressures that the chiropractors allege are responsible for disease do not exist. The present high
priest of chiropractic, B. J. Palmer, son of D. D.
Palmer, is a salesman *par excellence*. Salesmanship
and advertising are conspicuous in the chiropractic
curriculum. Palmer takes advantage of every opening. His latest device is a neurocalometer, which
makes even the apparatus of Abrams a trivial and
simple thing. The neurocalometer is put on the back
and presumably tells the chiropractor what bones

ought to be pushed back into place. Costing probably less than $50, it was originally leased to chiro-
practors at ten years for $626 and ultimately
brought as high as $2,500. The inordinate greed
of B. J. apparently incited revolt in the chiropractic
ménage and out of it. But the selling system and
the utter lack of any intelligence test for those entering the profession make it exceedingly popular
as a side-line to blacksmithing, pugilism, physical
culture and beauty shops. The complete story of
this great American medical folly may be found in
the earlier volume of this series.

Chirothesians. This peculiar group emanates
from California, its fountain head—the Western
College of Drugless Therapeutics. It combines a
new religious cult with medical hocus. Many state
laws give amnesty to religious healers. The cata-
logue of the college says: "While working under
this title healers ordained to work are protected from
annoyance by the state medical board." Evidently
a chirothesian is not limited to any system. One had
his office full of bottles labeled cancer, paralysis,
rheumatism and tumors; another said that he made
his diagnoses by examination of the pulse and "irido-
diagnosis." (For the latter system, see under "I.")
Chirothesianism is apparently a method of mixing
religion and fake healing to get around the medical
practice laws.

Christian Philosophers. The Christian Philosophical Institute, Wilbert LeRoy Casper, D. D., Ph.D., Bishop, holds forth in Oakland, Calif. It advertises health-happiness-prosperity, personally or by mail. Private treatments are $10 a month, group treatments by the Watch-Tower staff $1 a month. The first consultation is with "Dr. Casper who, for his own satisfaction, uses the Sixth Sense method of mental discernment in locating the patient's ailments." Casper plays the cult game clear across the board. He grants degrees of D. D. and C. P. in six months, conferring a beautiful diploma. The D. D. was $50; C. P., $100. He promoted a moving picture called the "Kingdom of Human Hearts." The lady who played the rôle of "Faith" sued him for $6,255 back salary as secretary and actress. In 1924 he went bankrupt, listing his assets as 12 collection boxes, 12 collection bottles, 11 boxes of posters and a painting eight feet square (value unknown). When he ran afoul of the law, testimony indicated his connection with certain osteopaths. He practiced obstetrics, endeavoring to conjure forth the child by dancing about, laying on hands and boisterous conduct generally.

Christian Science. Mary Baker Eddy was born in New Hampshire in 1821. From early life she showed all the characteristics of hysteria. At thirty-four years of age, she fell on the ice and developed an hysterical paralysis. When she was forty years old, she found Dr. P. P. Quimby, who cured her by means of ordinary psychotherapy. This she regarded as a divine revelation. Quimby, previously a watch maker, turned to mesmerism and from that developed his system of mental healing. When Mary Eddy met Quimby she learned his technique. After his death she started schools in Lynn, Mass., and later in Boston, to teach her methods. Besides charging her pupils a substantial fee she collected a royalty on their earnings after graduation. Her book, "Science and Health," first published in 1875, has had some 200 editions. Woodbridge Riley has proved that the scheme of Mrs. Eddy derived from three influences, "Shakerism," "Quimbyism" and "Alcott's Metaphysical System." Dresser has shown her direct plagiarism from Quimby's manuscripts and Peabody has revealed plagiarism from Alcott's writings.

Here is a system of healing which contends that suffering and death do not exist. It is a philosophy compounded of "vague maunderings about God, mind, matter, sin, disease, health, harmony, the denial of error" and similar topics. But as the great French psychiatrist, Janet, emphasizes, "It should not be forgotten that these vague and absurd utterances have succeeded in founding cathedrals and in comforting millions of men."

No doubt, persons with mental disease are benefited by mental treatment. But the records of cures furnished by Christian Scientists are a snare and a delusion. The diagnoses have been made by the patients themselves. After all, nature tends toward healing. The living cell wants to recover. All of the healing cults since time immemorial have floated themselves on this fact. In evaluating any method of healing allowance must be made for this *vis medicatrix naturæ*. But Christian Science healers do not allow for it; they claim they *are* it.

The growth of Eddyism has been a demonstration of what astute management can do for any healing system. The religious background makes it immune from legal prosecution. Mrs. Eddy's Boston school; the books and periodicals; the treatments, direct and absent, have yielded incalculable revenue. By her intense egoism, energy and unshakable belief in herself Mary Baker Eddy, thrice married, ultimately became sainted by her followers, endowed with a halo, and her cult is to-day almost immune from attack. The policy of intimidation and suppression and the verbal onslaughts of the Christian Science Committee on Publications have made the whole subject almost anathema to tired editors.

Christian Science is essentially the apotheosis of faith healing. Other systems preceded and have followed it. But the full glory of the blossom will perhaps never be visible again as in this specimen when at its best.

Even the name of this absurd cult is a misnomer. Its practitioners constantly fail to observe the golden rule, doing those whom they cannot be done by. If anything it is scientific, since the practice of absent treatment has reduced the art of living without apparent work to a science.

Christos (blood washers). A half-dozen cults use the term, "blood washing," as a come-on. It usually refers to some method of purging the intestinal tract. The Christos cult consists mostly of Negroes. Herb tonics are dispensed with the claim that they are especially blessed by Christ, the Savior. Taken in the form of tea, these herbs wash the blood of sin and impurities. New York authorities arrested and prosecuted the Negro leaders.

Chromopathy. Naturopathic physicians who practiced White's colored light system on the side used this term to indicate the healing of disease by colored lights.

Chromatherapy. Another modification of White's colored light scheme.

Couéism. Out of France, heralded by such exploitation as was never before given to the introduction of any new system of healing, came Emile Coué, druggist of Nancy. The system that he urged was "Self-Mastery by Conscious Auto-Suggestion." According to Coué, the power to control the activities of the body by auto-suggestion, is, like sin, an original endowment. Every human being possesses it at birth, and if one knows how to practice it consciously one may bring physical health to the sick, moral health to the neurotic and erring, and guide into right paths those who incline to dalliance along the primrose way.

Among the testimonials published by Coué and his followers were claims for the cure of organic heart disease, tuberculosis, asthma, prolapse of the uterus, hunchback, infection of the frontal sinus that had resisted eleven operations, paralysis of the limbs, club foot, bunions, varicose ulcer and practically everything that made anybody sick, anywhere, any time.

The method of M. Coué is simplicity itself. The patient is instructed as follows:

> Every morning before you are fully awake and every evening as soon as you are in bed, close your eyes and murmur twenty times: "Day by day in every way I'm getting better and better." It is well to be provided with a piece of string with twenty knots tied in it so that the counting may be mechanical. Let this auto-suggestion be made with confidence and with faith. The greater the confidence, the more rapid and certain the results. Further, each time, whether by day or by night, a physical and moral suffering is experienced, affirm instantly to yourself that you will not consciously encourage its existence and that you can make it disappear. Then, if possible, close your eyes and isolate yourself in thought, pass your hands lightly over the seat of pain, or on the forehead if the suffering be mental, and say as

quickly as possible aloud, as long as is necessary, "It's going."   On each recurrence of the
pain, employ the same method. These exercises
must be made with great simplicity and above
all without effort.

This is, of course, merely Christian Science with
reverse English. If the patient has a tumor of the
spinal cord, an infection of the heart or a cancer of
the stomach, and if he is under the care of a competent physician, he can do no harm by occupying his
spare moments in the mental exercises suggested.

When M. Coué himself conducted the cure the
procedure was much more elaborate. Then he emphasized to his people the functioning of every
organ, calling each by its name. The prophet
actually became lyrical. He told his patients that
they would sleep soundly, that their dreams would be
pleasant, that troubles and worries would melt away,
that they would awaken to sing, not sigh, that there
would be no more fears, no more thoughts of unkind-
ness, and that shyness and self-consciousness would
vanish. Above all, M. Coué assured the waiting
hundreds that the stomach and intestines would function regularly and copiously. So persuasive were
his words that the vice-provost of Eton related how,
at one of the séances, "hardly had M. Coué finished
speaking of the certain cure of constipation when the
sufferer he had been addressing hurried from the
room, announcing with mingled surprise and triumph

that the event was going to justify the prediction."
Truly words may move mountains!

Scientifically expressed the laws of M. Coué were:
When the will and the imagination are antagonistic,
the imagination always wins. In the conflict between
the will and the imagination the force of the imagination is in direct ratio to the square of the will. When
the will and the imagination are in one agreement,
one is multiplied by the other. The imagination
can be directed. To accept any of these laws as established, or as consistent with the established principles of psychology is quite impossible. Moreover,
they conflict with common sense and with the facts
of human disease as they have been established by
medical science.

So, M. Coué came to the United States, heralded
by newspaper publicity planned by a great syndicate,
whose managers should have known better. During
his tour he was featured by radio, by motion picture,
by lecture, and by all the other plans that the pub-
licists use for snaring the unwary.

The man himself gave an impression of sincerity
and childlike earnestness. He seemed genuinely
convinced of his own powers of healing and of the
fact that he had made a great contribution to medical science. Of the many cults built on faith healing
his was the first that had not been erected on a religious basis with more or less specific claims of
divine inspiration, and this, no doubt, was partially
responsible for its speedy tendency to oblivion. In

one of his meetings in Chicago an elderly woman, emaciated, feeble, short of breath and with every appearance of heart disease was urged, stimulated and encouraged to walk vigorously. Under the stimulus of the excitement she succeeded temporarily by the exercise of every reserve of energy, and after having served the purpose of this demonstration she retired from view, panting and exhausted. Later it was found that death had undoubtedly been hastened in several patients by this urging to activity which the weakened organs could not bear.

The atmosphere of a Coué demonstration was like that of a vaudeville hypnotist; the magic words, the mesmeric passes and even the old parlor trick of suggesting to members of the audience that they could not separate their hands after they had pressed them tightly together, were utilized to hold attention. And in the background were the crippled, the deformed and the disappointed dupes decoyed by the careless sensationalism of the press.

"M. Coué gave four performances at Orchestra Hall (in Chicago), seating about 3,700 persons, with a top price of $2.00," wrote Paul Leach. "On the one side of the footlights, 3,600 persons, there to see a new show, something different to please their appetites satiated with foxtrot dancing, cats and canaries, and Ziegfeld Follies. On the other side of the footlights, the man who earnestly tries to tell them all that he is no miracle worker; behind him more than one hundred cripples. Whether he cures some or not, I have a mental picture of a mother who sat in the front row on the stage, directly behind the man from Nancy, on her knees an eight-year-old boy whose eyes have never seen. The boy sat with bowed head, patiently, now and then twisting his slender fingers, an eager smile on his lips. He had been told he would be made to see.

"There come storms of applause from the other side of the footlights.

" 'What is it?' the blind boy asks eagerly.

" 'Some one has been cured,' he is told.

"Outside, half an hour later, the boy patiently asks why M. Coué did not make him see with his eyes that have never seen.

"On Saturday M. Coué sails for France, for Nancy. He will probably build himself a new château. Fifteen thousand persons at four Coué performances had a new thrill. The eight-year-old blind boy still sits patiently twisting long fingers and wondering why."

The Nancy to which M. Coué returned to quiet oblivion was the home of a school of scientific hypnotism, under the leadership of the great psychologists Liebeault and Bernheim, famous in the sixth and subsequent decades of the nineteenth century. The abrupt relief of hysterical symptoms by suggestion and persuasion is a commonplace in the practice of the average physician. Unconsciously it is used by

every successful doctor in the form of encourage-
ment and optimistic predictions of recovery. It is
the basis of the cult of healing brought to high
financial power by Mrs. Mary Baker Glover Eddy.
As long as there are fools to believe, it can always
be made the basis of a successful faith-healing cult.
And as long as there are men there will always be
believers.

Not long after Coué returned to France he died.
He left little of the funds he might have accumulated. Apparently the promoters had taken the
lion's share. And when the prophet dies, the cult
soon passes to purgatory with him, unless, as was
the case of Mary Baker Eddy, it has a financial
genius to arrange properly for its continuance.

D

Defensive Diet. G. E. Harter, Toledo, Ohio, is
responsible for the Defensive Diet League of America, annual dues, $10; associate membership, $5.
The fundamental principle is that "all so-called
diseases are but so many more or less localized
manifestations or symptoms—vents, safety-valves,
perhaps warnings at least—of one underlying condition, toxemia, the result of acidosis, brought about
by habitual and long continued eating of the wrong
foods at the wrong times or in wrong combinations."
He has adopted besides the views of half a dozen

other dietary faddists: He opposes the use of salt; he objects to eating fruits and starches at the same time; he urges three bowel actions daily; and he has much to say for sauerkraut. His original association with a periodical devoted to dentistry made him pick the dentists as his first victims in promoting his scheme. Mr. Harter is no authority on diet and those whom he cites as authorities have been known for years as the exponents of peculiar dietary fads.

Among the authorities cited by Harter—in defense of his Defensive Diet—are J. H. Tilden, who for some years conducted a so-called health school and ran as an advertising medium a small magazine called the *Stuffed Club*. Later Tilden expanded this to a school of healing and named his periodical the *Philosophy of Health*. Harter calls Tilden "the head of the dietetic profession in America, probably in the world." This tender compliment is bound to be a great blow to such experts as McCollum, Hindhede and the professors of digestive science in our great medical schools.

The blah associated with Harter's efforts is sufficient to convict him of folly even were the jury to be composed of readers of Macfadden's *Physical Culture*. "Disease is due to toxemia," he says. Then he urges that toxemia is due to enervation and enervation is due to improper eating. He assures his followers that tuberculosis is not due to a germ, that smallpox is not contagious and that the "germ theory" is "merely a plausible fallacy."

At the first annual meeting of the directors of his league Mr. Harter explained his campaign with the following touching tribute to his own powers:

"Last year and every year a half million people died and are dying for lack of the knowledge I can give them . . . and another half million little helpless children, between the ages of six and ten, are dying every year because I have not told their parents the things that I know about the food they eat."

Harter also had for sale bulletins on diet, a "Dietetic Baking Powder," a food chart, a steam-pressure cooker and a fruit and vegetable press.

Of all the fads promoted in our land the dietary fads are most numerous. They run from starvation to special diets containing everything that one might eat modified in every possible way. Harter is not the first to exploit these dietary misconceptions for personal gain.

Divine Science. Treatment of illness by "Divine Science" consists in persuading the sufferer that God is good, that disease is the result of man's own foolishness and that God will cure him if he will give him a chance. These simple doctrines are shrouded, however, in the usual preposterous verbosity. Faith is secured by prayer, with the laying on of hands. The followers of Dowie, Schlatter,

Newell, Hickson, Voliva, and more recently John Murray, are the chief disciples of this school of healing.

Dowieism. About 1900 Alexander Dowie announced that he was the prophet Elijah returned to earth, although without a chariot. He healed by the laying on of hands. His system was obviously faith healing. As a promoter Dowie was no doubt second only to Mrs. Eddy in this country. He built up a large following, established a city with tremendous industries and established church observances and ritual sufficient to occupy the minds of those who followed him. Like other prophets of healing he thundered against physicians and attacked preventive vaccination. When he passed on, the holy robes succeeded to Glenn Wilbur Voliva, now the czar of Zion City, the Jerusalem of the cult. Voliva thinks the world is flat.

E

Eclecticism. Among physicians who treat disease by drugs it has been customary to include the regular medical profession (allopaths), the homeopathic, eclectic and physio-medical groups. About 1800 scientific medicine was undergoing a period of revolt against the giving of drugs which had drastic action. Homeopathy (see later) and eclecticism owed much of their initial success, no doubt, to the fact that they prescribed milder remedies which at least did not interfere with the natural tendency of the body toward recovery. Eclecticism discarded mineral drugs and emphasized the use of plant remedies for specific conditions. It urged the use of single remedies and most simple combinations. For a complete story of its rise and fall see the account elsewhere in this volume.

Eddyism.   See Christian Science.

Electric Light Diagnosis and Therapy.   See Electrotherapy.

Electro-Homeopathy.   A combination of electrotherapy and homeopathy.   (See under each.)

Electro-Naprapathy.   A combination of two cults.   (See under each.)

Electronic Therapy.   Albert Abrams departed this life in 1924.   For a brief span of years the system that he devised for diagnosing disease and for treating such conditions as he diagnosed caught the fancy of numerous followers, bewildered the ignorant, and amazed even hardened investigators by its superlative chicanery.   Of his original system of spondylotherapy more will be said later.   Electronic medicine embraces the following procedure: One secures from a prospective patient a drop of

blood upon a piece of filter paper. This is put in
an apparatus called a dynamizer, which in turn is
connected with a rheostatic dynamizer from which
wires pass to a vibratory rheostat which is finally
connected with a measuring rheostat from which a
wire passes to the forehead of some available subject, quite healthy and employed at a small salary.
This person faces west in a dim light. An obliging
assistant turns the switch and the electronic therapist thumps on the abdomen of the subject. Abrams
insisted that varying areas of dullness in the subject's abdomen connoted various diseases in the persons contributing the blood. On this basis he devised an apparatus called the oscilloclast for treating
such persons with appropriate vibrations. He
claimed the ability to tell the religion of the person
submitting the blood and to diagnose disease by
this method from the handwriting.

The Abrams system included the complete scheme
of quackery: A special association, a special periodical, a school, traveling lectureships, leasing of
apparatus with a contract not to open it, and constant charges of persecution against investigators.

On his death, Abrams left an estate of more than
a million dollars; his executors continue to promote
the cult in San Francisco. But the handwriting on
the wall indicates that the cult lacks the master
hand of its egocentric leader. Abramism is to be
credited with the most rapid and conspicuous rise

and fall of any cult of our modern period. (See also the complete history in the previous volume.)

Electrotherapy. The use of electric devices has a definite place in the treatment of disease. It should not be thought, however, that any electrician or machinist is competent to use such methods. Electricity is a two-edged sword; in the hands of the ignorant, it may wreak disaster. Actually its use should be limited to those who have had the training of a physician and then given special study to the use of electric devices or to competent technicians working under the direction of a physician.

Emmanuel Movement. In 1906 the Emmanuel Church Health Class was organized by Dr. Elwood Worcester and Dr. Samuel McComb, rector of Emmanuel Church, an Episcopalian church in Boston. It was planned perhaps as a resisting movement to Eddyism, with a view to combining the knowledge of a physician and the influence of the church in the healing of nervous and mental diseases. The movement spread; other churches were established and books were sold in profusion. As long as it is limited to the mental conditions Emmanuelism probably does little harm. One wonders how far it substitutes a religious interest for some underlying mental habit that is responsible for the illness and that ought to be removed. How

far does it fail by overlooking organic causes of
mental disease?

Erosionism.   See McLean.

F

Faith Healing.   Records may be found in all re-
ligions from the earliest times of remarkable cures
resulting from faith, grace, inspiration, prayer, con-
version or what not.   Obviously these do not concern organic disease that has been subjected to
scientific diagnosis.   Such cures constitute the very
elements of all of the systems of healing based on a
single idea as to the cause and cure of disease.   Essentially the manifestations concerned are to be
studied as psychologic phenomena.   The ancient
Greek, Hebrew and Egyptian physicians used faith-
healing methods as a part of their combinations of
priesthood and physicianship.   The Druid priests
and Indian medicine men were thoroughly conversant with the powers of suggestion.   Mesmer and
animal magnetism yielded the host of faith-healing
cults which obtrude themselves upon us to-day.   As
has been shown, Phineas Quimby was conversant
with mesmerism.   From him Mrs. Eddy derived,
and, succeeding her, were New Thought, the Emmanuel movement; Mrs. Henry Milmans, Francis
Schlatter, the "Reverend" Charles F. McLean, the

Fire-Baptized Holiness Association; the Peculiar People, the Holiness Society of West Virginia, the Pennsylvania Hexen Charms; the Metaphysical Healers, the Mind Curists; the Viticulturists; the Magnetic Healers; the Phrenopathists; the Esoteric Vibrationists; the Occultists; the Venopathists; the Psychic Scientists; Couéism; much of psycho-analysis and most of psychotherapy. Besides, much of the alleged success of chiropractic, osteopathy and other methods of healing by the laying on of hands depends largely on the power of persuasion or faith healing.

What happens when the faith-healing methods are put to the crucial test of follow-up methods such as are now employed by large medical clinics to test the results of new methods? In May, 1923, evangelistic meetings with faith healing were held in Vancouver. Later the General Ministerial Association of Vancouver appointed a committee of ministers, doctors, university professors and one lawyer to look into the end results of the alleged cures. The evangelist refused to coöperate but the committee succeeded nevertheless in obtaining the names of three hundred and fifty persons who were presumably cured by his methods. The diseases included cancer, pyorrhea, epilepsy, bronchitis, neurasthenia, idiocy and some fifty-five others. Of all the patients only five were so benefited that they might be called cures at the end of six months. Thirty-eight patients showed general improvement, but two hundred and twelve declared cured after anointing were found unchanged and seventeen were distinctly worse. Thirty-nine of the cured patients were dead after six months. Five of the persons anointed and four members of the families of anointed persons were found in institutions for the insane. Of the five cases admittedly cured all were in the group classified by sound diagnosticians as nervous or mental diseases. They included a girl who stammered before and had not stammered since; an hysterical paralytic who merely had convinced herself that she was paralyzed and who was unconvinced after the anointing; a confirmed invalid who enjoyed a variety of ill-health, including many ailments, but whose physicians called her hysterical; a man who had diagnosed his own condition as "internal goiter" without consulting a physician. The lump he thought he felt in his throat disappeared promptly after the anointing. Doctors call this condition "globus hystericus."

G

Geotherapy. New York investigators found a concern treating disease by the application of little pads of earth—hence the grandiloquent title. A warning resulted in the abandonment of the enterprise.

Gland Therapy. Within recent years no method

of treating disease has aroused more interest than has glandular therapy. The use of products such as insulin from the pancreatic gland; thyroid extract from the thyroid gland; adrenalin from the adrenal gland; pituitary extract from the pituitary gland, and most recently, of parathyrin from the parathyroid glands, is based on sound scientific observation. The treatment of glandular deficiencies by supplying the missing elements seems to be limited thus far largely to those that have been mentioned. In the case of the sex glands, deficiencies seem to be relieved in some instances by transplantations which survive over varying periods of time. However, in no field of medicine to-day is such far-reaching imposition practiced as in the giving of doses of mixed gland preparations and of preparations of single glands, not established as of any real value, for the treatment of all sorts of disorders. This polyglandular therapy has in many instances almost assumed the proportions of a cult.

H

Homeopathy. In 1810, Samuel Christian Hahnemann presented to the world the homeopathic bible. His system of disease and its healing involved three main tenets, the chief of which is embodied for posterity in the phrase "similia similibus curantur," a phrase which contends that disease or symptoms of disease are curable by particu-

lar drugs which produce similar effects on the
healthy body. The cult thrived on the weaknesses
of the so-called regular medical practice of its period.
When scientific medicine began to discard overdoses
of too potent drugs and to rely on medicaments of
proved value, homeopathy dwindled into its present
state of moribundity. During 1925 there were
forty-nine homeopathic graduates, and it seems safe
to predict that another generation will see the
complete passing of this offshoot of regular medicine. Its great folly was the dilution of drugs to a
point at which one might just as well have administered the water of Lake Erie, or if it were not
for the salt, of the Pacific Ocean. Hahnemann and
Homeopathy are also fully considered in "The
Medical Follies."

I

Irido-Diagnosis. The poetical notion that the
eye is the mirror of the soul evidently convinced a
minor medical prophet in Chicago that money might
be made by founding a school of medicine in which
the diagnosis of all diseases would depend on the
ability to notice the changing colors of the iris or
colored material of the eye. With a remarkable
genius for publicity, he succeeded in attracting much
free newspaper mention and in leading to his school
numerous ignorant satellites who desired to enter
on the practice of healing by some easy route.

Among those attracted have been a few regularly licensed physicians who sought to exploit themselves and enhance their incomes by adding the claim of this superior power to such as might already have been conferred upon them by the state. Even to-day the practitioners of this vagary burst into temporary luminescence in the sensation-seeking press. Fortunately the prophet himself was accused by his wife of mental vagaries. He gradually subsides!

J

Jewish Science. Rabbi Morris Lichtenstein, perhaps somewhat jealous of the profits of Christian Science, prepared a book of "Jewish Science and Health" with all of the orotund verbosity of the work which he affected to simulate. He established an elaborate ritual of prayers, a health prayer consisting of two parts: First, the visualization of divine giving and then of man's receiving the process of healing and the state of health restored through that process. If any particular organ of the body is affected, the prayer must affirm that health is saturating and obliterating all defection and suffering.

K

Kneipp Cure. See Naturopathy.

L

Leonic Healers. A group of colored mystics established themselves in New York City and advertised their healing powers under the signs of the Zodiac, offering at the same time horoscopic service and direction. The authorities believing the "Leonic healers" to be more "lyin'" than Leonic, arrested the group and secured the assessment of small fines in municipal courts. The enterprise was shortly abandoned.

Limpio Comerology. A Mrs. Caroline M. Olsen and her husband, Emil, hailing from St. Louis, adopted the name of Limpio Comerology for their health service, which appears to have been founded primarily on the doctrine of clean eating. In connection with the teaching of the science, there were dispensed "Q-33" and "Q-34," proprietary preparations, to make the clean eating physically successful. Mrs. Olsen, obviously Norwegian or Danish, explained that the term "Limpio Comerology" was taken from the Spanish.

M

McFerrin. Upon the programs of women's clubs that like to indulge themselves in free lectures, regardless of the truth or quality of the lecturer, one "Dr." Charles B. McFerrin, "Food Scientist, Diet Specialist, Humorist," is a not infrequent feature. He also gives courses at $15 each.

McFerrin is a follower of Eugene Christian, Alsaker, Macfadden, Brinkler and Tilden. He thinks that the combining of stewed tomatoes and creamed or mashed potatoes has a strong tendency to tear up the mucous lining of the stomach and intestines, causing constipation and a general acid or sour condition of the body, making asthma, nervousness, rheumatism or other maladies possible. For this sweet thought there is not, of course, the slightest evidence.

Like most cultists with one-idea systems as to the causation and cure of disease McFerrin insists that all disease is due to malnutrition. He promotes also, however, a system of breathing exercises under the title "The Rhythmic or Success Breath," and he urges for almost every ailment to which flesh may be heir, prolonged soaking in water of a temperature the same as that of the body. According to his assertion, after three hours in the tub "the water penetrates the internal organs in a manner floating them and relieving much pressure on each other," while in from six to nine hours "the liver is wonderfully purified" and "gall stones many times soften and pass away with ease, thus saving an expensive and painful operation." This absolutely proves the status of Charles B. McFerrin as a humorist, since no claim seems to be too funny for him to try it.

A long list of services that may be rendered and of the various prices for them is the tragical antithesis, proving that the matter of getting the money is a serious business if not a science.

McLean. James A. M. McLean, born in Martinique, claims that he is a geologist, evolutionist, pathologist, psychologist, anatomist, biologist, chemist, erosionist and theophonist. Like many other quacks, he turned up in California, claiming in his advertisements the special powers of reducing and building up obesity, and reducing various disorders, diseases and infirmities. His system was a combination of physical, metaphysical and spiritual healing—bunk from start to finish.

Mysticism. Practically all of the cults relying on faith healing and suggestion adopt forms of mysticism in order to exploit to the utmost the credulous belief in magic. Such healing formed the basis of cabalistic incantations and necromancy of the church healings of the Middle Ages and of the spiritualistic wizardry of our modern times. The fear of the powers of the unknown and the will to believe in fairies and demons beyond the age of adolescence are the pabulum on which mystic cults of healing thrive.

N

Naprapathy. According to the statement of Dr. Oakley Smith, founder and president of the Chicago College of Naprapathy, the chief tenet of that school is the belief that nerve function is impaired by the contraction of the connective tissue through which the nerves pass. "Naprapathy teaches that the real disease is in the shrunken ligament, and the conditions in the body heretofore believed to be the disease are but the symptoms of the real disease in the ligament, the 'ligatight,' the predisposing cause." Of course, this cult believes that drugs and surgery in the treatment of diseased ligaments are not only useless but are harmful. The Chicago institution was founded in 1908 and moved about from one old house to another until it occupied a three-story building in 1910.

With the cleaning up of medical practice in Illinois, this institution found the going difficult, as did many others. Obviously an offshoot of chiropractic, it teaches that the contracted ligaments are cured not by adjusting the vertebra of the spine, but by using the vertebræ as levers to stretch the ligaments. The present year finds the college still existing, but obviously of little moment as compared with the cults that attract their thousands to naprapathy's hundreds.

Naturology. This is merely another name for

naturopathy. This school was founded by a naturopath of the Benedict Lust school who adopted this fanciful name to show that he knew things that even they didn't know.

Naturopathy. According to legislation proposed in Connecticut, naturopathy means the practice of psychologic, medical and material sciences of healing; including the psychologic sciences such as psychotherapy; the medical sciences such as medicotherapy, articular manipulation, massage, corrective and orthopedic gymnastics, neurotherapy, physiotherapy, hydrotherapy, electrotherapy, thermotherapy, phototherapy, chromotherapy, divisilotherapy, pneumotherapy and zonotherapy; and the material sciences such as dietetics, histology therapy and external applications, but shall not be held to mean internal medication.

Obviously here is a medical cesspool with legislation planned to give opportunity to every form of healing that departs from regular medicine. The main school of naturopathy is operated by one B. Lust, N.D. This institution, the American School of Naturopathy, issues diplomas showing that its graduates have honorably passed the examination in full regarding naturologic and naturopathic courses.

The publication of the cult was for many years the "Herald of Health," which was a sales manual not only for the peculiar devices and literary documents promoted by the fountain head, but also for all of the peculiar medical nostrums of healing which form the stock in trade of irresponsible faddists. The early issues of this publication promote dozens of dietary fallacies, fasting, hot and cold water systems, milk systems, scientific relaxation, exercise, health resorts, magnetic healing, mud packs, vegetarian and fruitarian diets and.what not. The outlet to-day for these faddists is the publishing plant of Bernarr Macfadden.

Mr. Lust's own definition of naturopathy includes the "art of natural healing and the science of physical and mental regeneration on the basis of self-reform, natural life, clean and normal diet, hydrotherapy (Paiessnitz, Kneipp, Lehmann and Just system), osteopathy, chiropractic, naturotherapy, electrotherapy (sunlight and air cult), diet, phytotherapy, physical and mental culture to the exclusion of poisonous drugs and non-adjustable surgery." There is the system in a nutshell, and what an irrational nut it is. In a word, naturopathy is the capitalization for purposes of financial gain of the old advice that outdoor living, good diet and enough exercise and rest are conducive to health and longevity. When these simple principles can be linked with the sale of worthless pamphlets, intricate apparatus or faith cures, the formulas yield gold.

New Thought. The term "New Thought"

covers the teaching of all of the modern healing cults, including Christian Science and Jewish Science. It is, however, promoted through the "National New Thought Society" and the "International New Thought Alliance." Its legitimate predecessor was the "Transcendental Movement" of 1830, and is influenced by the doctrines of reincarnation and telepathy. Numerous teachers give lectures on relaxation, visualization, accomplishment and manifestation, and activities with music, rhythmic exercise, "vitalic" breathing and similar bunk. Hindus, and Senegambians costumed like Hindus, have their followers in centers of Yogi philosophy and mysticism. At the last annual convention, ten thousand dreamers were present. The "New Thought" bible is Ralph Trine's book, "In Tune with the Infinite," which has passed through seven hundred editions.

O

Orificial Therapy.   The strange notion that the majority of human complaints result from pressure and insufficient relaxation of the various openings out of and into the human body made Dr. E. H. Pratt of Chicago the founder and minor prophet of another cult. The enthusiasm with which he promoted this extraordinary doctrine led to him the usual strollers on the paths of medical fallacy. It is pitiful to cogitate on the surgical sins committed in the name of this cult. Its followers to-day number not more than a few hundred. The treatment of disease of the various orifices by scientific methods is, of course, a part of all medicine.

Osteopathy. On June 22, 1874, Andrew Still, a freelance doctor among the Shawnee Indians in Kansas, flung to the breezes the banner of osteopathy. Convinced of the fact that this system of healing was a divine revelation, and being of a somewhat medical turn of mind, he planned a system of healing based on manipulations and adjustments. Since his time, earnest osteopaths have attempted to make the cult evolve into something approaching scientific medicine with a view to giving it permanence. Unfortunately, it must be considered as merely a backdoor entrance into the practice of healing. It wanes constantly before the onslaught of chiropractic, the outgrowth itself of osteopathy, and of actual scientific medicine, which is not dependent on folly. Osteopathy also is considered elaborately in "The Medical Follies."

P

Pathiatry. This particular cult is trade-marked. "It combines the best principles of spinal adjustment, traction, manipulation, deep massage, etc., administered by oneself. So simple and delightful as to become a part of the daily toilet. Done anywhere, at any time, while standing, even sitting; without appliance of any kind."

Poropathy. Arthur de Collard turned up in Richmond, Va., and persuaded the legislature in that State, in 1918, to license him to practice poropathy. Arthur claimed to be a cousin of Napoleon and a graduate of several European universities. His diplomas, he said, had all been burned, and he would not answer the simplest question on the elements of medicine and surgery. The bill defined poropathy and manipulative surgery as a new branch of therapeutics. It employs no medicine taken through the stomach and does not employ the knife. Healing and curative agencies and lotions, however, applied directly to the diseased organs and to the nerves controlling those organs, through the pores of the skin and mucous membrane, which are opened by medical manipulation, immediately reach the disease or ailment through the eliminating organs, and by this process heal and cure most of the ills to which flesh is heir, including: internal cancer, cerebrospinal meningitis, epilepsy, tuberculosis of the joints and heart disease. This system, according to the bill, would adjust, heal and cure broken bones, sprains and dislocations. After a committee substitute for the bill and various amendments to the substitute had been rejected, the bill was passed and Arthur de Collard through it acquired the right to practice poropathy in Virginia. There are now several poropathists in the state who have taken a course under de Collard.

Practo-therapy. This was a group of men and women, mostly nurses, who treated human ills through intestinal irrigation, "Practo-therapy" evidently being a fanciful title in place of the word "procto."

Q

Quartz-therapy. This included a group of "Naturopath" irregulars who use Krohmayer lamps in their business. The Krohmayer lamp provides ultraviolet rays which pass through quartz but not through ordinary glass.

R

Rawson's School. F. S. Rawson founded a school in 1919, which works on the negative rather than on the positive principle. The person is supposed to deny vehemently again and again the thing that he does not want. Obviously, this also is Christian Science with reverse English. Some hundred practitioners find it commercially successful.

S

Sanatology. Sanatology is a delightful title conferred on his particular science of healing by Dr. P.
L. Clark, Chicago, who insists that he is the first
man in the world to make the pronouncement and
prove that acidosis and toxicosis are the two basic
causes of all disease. In his school on Prairie Ave-
nue in Chicago he teaches people, so he says, how
to remove the causes and restore the body to normal.
He issues little cards for free consultation and
blood-pressure test, which are the "come-ons" by
which he secures permanent contributors.

Scientific Christianity. With headquarters in
Kansas City, this organization publishes *Unity,*
with a circulation of 185,000. It sends out lec-
turers, organizes communities, maintains prayer
services, reaching some three to five million people
yearly, not counting its recent attempts on the radio.
The periodical is full of the usual preposterous
testimonials of too credulous victims. A lady in
Hot Springs sends a tithe of $50 because a hail-
storm passed over her front yard. The funds come
from tithings of 10 per cent. The headquarters in
New York is directed by Mr. Richard Lynch, who
talks on health, happiness, prosperity and character
formation to from three hundred to five hundred
people. In 1923, he had an audience of six. He

has probably, however, reached his maximum growth.

Somapathy. The Illinois College of Somapathy is located at Elgin, Illinois, and its fond father is Dr. C. H. Murray. It appears that this science is devoted to the body suffering. The diagnostician feels around in the place where the nerves emerge from the spinal cord and adjusts them. Then he continues his good effects by applying ice cold, or material heated up to two hundred degrees at the place of adjustment. Here again is an offshoot of chiropractic and osteopathy, with which it is associated in another school. Dr. Murray promises his graduates $10,000 a year if they are successful.

Spectrocromists. This was an establishment operated through advising individuals to wear clothing or garments according to the color of the spectrum. How they came to the conclusion as to what part of the spectrum the individual should assume, in selecting his colors, is not clear. Perhaps it was for this advice they charged. They have been arrested and fined.

Spiritualism. Houdini exposed spiritualism so successfully that only the most credulous are likely to believe in its healing virtues. The beliefs that insanity is due to the poisons of evil spirits and that the ghosts of famous physicians are able to write prescriptions through a medium are so absurd as to merit hardly a moment's attention. Dr. Titus Bull in New York maintains that he has the power to heal by driving out evil spirits through his own saintliness and by the laying on of hands. The idea that there can be anything saintly in this laying on of hands, in the vernacular of the day, is Titus' "bull."

T

Telathermy. A former adherent of Abrams' electronic fraud improved on it by developing a box or contrivance with a vibrator which was supposed to increase the number of vibrations and become louder when certain reactions were expected from certain dupes undertaking this treatment. Joslin, now of Chicago, formerly of Riverside Drive, New York City, was one of the operators of this apparatus. When the health officials raided the place, they found the apparatus to consist of a vibrating armature of an electric call bell, with a small battery hidden in a secret recess in the lower part of the box. As the patient placed the box on his lap or on his chest, the weight of the apparatus would make a contact which would cause the armature to vibrate. Pressure of the operator on the box would make a better connection and the vibration would be more constant and louder. The boss was arrested and fined.

Theophonism.   See McLean.

Theosophy.   Theosophy embodies telepathy and spiritualism with health interests somewhat secondary.   Nevertheless, much is made of the ability to produce relaxation and relief of pain by earnest prayer, a sort of "spiritual anesthetic."   A church mission of healing in New York, using this cult, is carried on by the Rev. Thomas Calvert, who has developed his own system of psychoanalysis and complexes, and who will put them to work at $5 for forty-five minutes, $10 for ninety minutes, or $15 for two hours.

One Dr. John D. Quackenbos, with the accent on the first syllable of the last name, claimed that he has cured more than twenty thousand cases of drug addiction by a system of mental maneuvers, associated with metaphysical healing.

Tropo-therapy.   This was a group of food faddists advertising special nutritional foods under this fanciful name.

V

Vita-O-Pathy.   The name of this particular system indicates how hopeless is any attempt to simplify the control of quackery.   Its prophet, Orrin Robertson, Ph.D., D.M., M.D., announces that:

Vita-O-Pathy is the essence and quintessence of the following thirty-six systems with additional discoveries and inventions; yet it is unlike any of them. Consequently it Restores Health to Humanity without a Surgical Operation. It is based on Geometry, a true science which contains the fundamental secrets of Ancient Science, Philosophy and Religion.

1 *Prana-Yama*
2 *Zoism*
3 *Spiritual Science*
4 *Psychic Sarcology*
5 *Somnopathy*
6 *Christian Science*
7 *Osteopathy*
8 *Chiropathy*
9 *Divine Science*
10 *Botanic*
11 *Allopathy*
12 *Biopneuma*
13 *Prayer Cure*
14 *Rest Cure*
15 *Diet Cure*
16 *Eclecticism*
17 *Hydropathy*
18 *Magnetism*
19 *Phrenopathy*
20 *Nervauric Therapeutics*
21 *Electro-Therapeutics*
22 *Chromopathy*
23 *Vitapathy*
24 *Homeopathy*
25 *Psychopathy*
26 *Magnetic Massage*

27 *Faith Cure*
28 *Biochemic System*
29 *Therapeutic Sarcognomy*
30 *Physio Medical*
31 *Mechanical Therapy*
32 *Suggestive Therapeutics*
33 *Auto-Suggestion*
34 *Tripsis*
35 *Spondylotherapy*
36 *Chirothesia*

He has worked out a scheme of muddling the moronic mind, and there are apparently enough persons of an intelligence below that of a child of eight to provide him with plenty of victims. His price varies from $40 a week to whatever he can get. It appears that he was born on May 28, 1858, in Cass County, Missouri, under the control of Archangel Haniel, who it seems controls Friday, and whose chief characteristic is spiritual love. Further than this the deponent saith not.

Z

Zodiac Therapy. This group was an offspring, formerly employed in an establishment called "Aero-therapy-Astral Healers." On the walls of the establishment, on blue paper, were photographic enlargements of signs of the Zodiac. The ceiling was painted to look like the heavens. Persons desiring their horoscope read, the effect of the horoscope on their health was determined, for which a charge was made. Pamphlets were sold, also herb remedies.

Zonotherapy. One Dr. Fitzgerald of Hartford, Connecticut, has divided the body into zones, lengthwise and crosswise, and heals disease in one zone by pressing on others. To keep the pressure going he developed little wire springs. For instance, a toothache on the right side may be "cured" by fastening a little spring around the second toe of the left foot. Naturally, Fitzgerald has never convinced any one with ordinary reasoning powers that there is anything in his system—except what he gets out of it.

CHAPTER II

THE CULT OF BEAUTY

I

In the classified telephone directory of any large American city one comes casually on the heading Barber Colleges, and proceeds then through Barbers, Baths and Beauty Culture Schools to Beauty Parlors. Then one advances to Corsets and Accessories, to Cosmeticians and to Dermatologists—and begins to realize at last what a vast trade has grown out of the desires of Mr. Babbitt and his wife and daughters to enhance the physiognomies and figures with which a none too beneficent Providence endowed them. If one resides in a town in which the trade is backward, the promoters of comeliness may still be found under such old-fashioned headings as Hair-dressers, but where the cult of beauty has many shrines they hold forth in all the gaudy glory of Beauticians and Cosmetologists.

As with classifications, so with names. In all of the cities in which the beauty shops flourish their sign-boards display an extraordinary similarity. Consider these samples plucked from several lists:

> Annie Laurie Beauty Parlor
> Bellcano Beauty College
> Bertha Betty Beauty-Spot Shop

Betty Jane Beauty Shoppe
Bonita Beauty Salon
Fountain-o'-Youth
Hollyd Obesity Salon (The first word is a
    contraction of Hollywood)
Babe's Beauty Shoppe
Beau Ideal Shoppe
Brush-Up Shop
Brownatone Shop
Char-Ming Beauty Shoppe
Colton's Permanent Wave Shop
The Fairest Marcel Shop
Franco-American Beauty Shop
Gotthart's Vienna Beauty Shop
Hindu Rose Beauty Parlor
Jean's System of Beauty
La-Ann Beauty Shop
La-Blanche Beauty Salon
Ladifair Shop
Maison Gustav
Maison de Sadie
Miladi Beauty Shop
Mi-Lady's Beauty Shop
Mitzi Beauty Shoppe
Paradise Beauty Shop
Madam Pauline
Peacock Beauty Shoppes
Poudre Box Beauty Shoppe
Premier Epilation Salon
Sanitary Beauty Parlor
Venus Beauty Parlor
Your Style Beauty Shop

Here are parlors, colleges, shops, shoppes and
salons, all conjuring with the magic word beauty

and conducted by damsels variously yclept, whose names have undergone strange metamorphoses in accordance with the nature of their art. Here are Eva May, Emmie Lou, Frances Jeune, Helen Janice, Kathryn Ann, Beatrix, Elza, Cecile, Cecille, Ethyle Clair, Sadye, Ada Dolores, Estelle, Mae, Gladys, Gloria, Hazelle, Helyn, Hannette, Myrtle, Jean Jonnie, Georgette, Arline, Kathlyn, Adoline, Marjorine and Neoma.

Proceeding through the telephone book, one reaches the heading Plastic Surgery, and comes upon the names of five or six medicos who, it seems, devote themselves to the removal of the redundant wrinkle, to restoring the aquilinity of misshaped proboscises, to the disposal of the fat resultant from too many calories, and to the miscellaneous alteration of countenances which, for one reason or another, seem to their possessors to be not what they ought to be. These learned gentry are obviously not to be listed with the ladies above mentioned, except in so far as they are also concerned with the glorification of American womanhood and womanlike manhood. Of their arts and their deceits more will be said later.

Estimates place the number of beauty shops in Manhattan at between fifteen hundred to two thousand. There are at least a thousand in Los Angeles, not counting Hollywood. The number in Florida increases with every incoming train, for the beauty shop, like the fur store, the jewelry store, the dance hall and the homes of "ladies of leisure," is among the first to profit when money is loose, profits are large and the turnover rapid. The high potentate of one college for cosmeticians informs me that nine thousand emporiums are devoted exclusively to the sale and application of her wares, and that an average of ten more or less sightly young women dispense beauty and its accessories at each of them. The casual trade in powders, soaps, creams, lotions, beauty masks, nose-shapers, chin-lifters, ear-pressers, hair-restorers, hair-removers, hair-straighteners and hair-tonics is a matter of millions.

Indeed, it is largely on their sale—they are endowed with names as fanciful as those of the ladies who promote them—that the beauty shop industry has arisen. All the rest of the hocus-pocus—the "colleges" for the training of apprentices, the various mysterious techniques and maneuvers, and the trade associations and their carefully planned publicity—are intended mainly to promote the traffic in toilet preparations. If one turns from that section in the telephone book devoted to beauty parlors and hair-dressers to that headed Cosmetics or Toilet Preparations, certain names will be found recurring with the significant words "manufacturing company" behind them. The company with the nine thousand dispensatories of cosmetic art manufactures one hundred and thirty-seven preparations. Corresponding to the Beau Ideal Shop we have the Beau Ideal Preparations, to the Boncilla Shops the

Boncilla Laboratories, Inc., to the Cara Mia Shops the Cara Mia, Inc., to the Charm of Youth Shops the Charm of Youth Corporation, to the Marinello Shops the Marinello Company. And so on through the list, with the independent ladies who conduct individual shops or parlors, perhaps in their own homes, supplied by manufacturers who deal in the various preparations in bulk. The business increases by leaps and bounds, and is acquiring a legal status. Let us cease for a moment these generalizations and gaze upon some concrete facts.

2

Arkansas, Connecticut, Illinois, Louisiana, Missouri, New Mexico, Oregon, Utah and Wisconsin are already in the fold with State licenses for beauticians, and the way is open in California, Texas, Oklahoma, Michigan, Iowa, Nebraska and New Hampshire.

In Illinois one cannot practice beauty culture without a certificate of registration as a beauty culturist. "Any one or any combination of the following practices constitutes the practice of beauty culture when done for cosmetic or beautifying purposes and not for the treatment of disease or of muscular or nervous disorder," says the law. Here, indeed, is a fine distinction, and the specifications go on to convey suggestions titillating to an active imagination. Beauty culture, according to the act, is "the application of cosmetic preparations to the human body by massaging, stroking, kneading, slapping, tapping, stimulating, manipulating, exercising, cleansing, beautifying, or by means of devices, apparatus or appliances, arranging, dressing, marcelling, curling, waving, cleansing, singeing, bleaching, coloring, dyeing, tinting, or otherwise treating by any means the hair of any person." I have seen a photograph of the governor of this proud State as he signed the law, his cranium, quite devoid of hirsutage, glowing beneath the countenance of an inspired cosmetician, who breathlessly awaits the application to the paper of the tintorial fluid that is to legalize her noble profession. But wait! Another great profession also pleads for protection! "However," says the act, "provisions of this act shall not authorize any registered beauty culturist to cut or clip the hair of any person unless he has first obtained a certificate of registration as a *barber*."

The law specifies who may be a registered apprentice in the art and limits the certificate of cosmetician to those who are at least sixteen years of age, of good moral character and temperate habits, and who have graduated from an eighth-grade elementary school or completed an equivalent course, and finally, who have either studied beauty culture for one year as registered apprentices or graduated from an approved school. Naturally, the legislators provided for admitting into the fold, pronto and without examination, all those who were practicing one year before the law was passed. Also they provided for the revocation of licenses for immorality, habitual drunkenness, gross malpractice, incompetency, continued practice by persons having contagious diseases, drug addiction and unprofessional conduct.

The Arkansas bill specifically mentions the removal of superfluous hair as a part of the cosmetic therapist's art. The Missouri law speaks of hairdressers, cosmeticians or cosmetologists as well as of beauty culturists. It also employs the words "cosmetology" and "cosmetological establishment." In its definition of the practices concerned it mentions particularly the removal of superfluous hair by electricity and speaks of the "limited practice of cosmetology" as the "occupation of manicurists and electrologists." The Missouri law requires the registration of each cosmetological establishment for purposes of sanitary control and bars the use of its rooms at any time for sleeping or residential purposes. It carefully exempts from the law members of the following liberal professions: medicine, surgery, dentistry, osteopathy, chiropody and barbering.

In Oregon the law takes another turn: there cosmetic therapy includes "the application of the hands or of mechanical or electric apparatus with or without cosmetic preparations, tonics, lotions, creams or clays, to massage, cleanse, stimulate, manipulate, exercise or otherwise improve or beautify the scalp, face, neck, shoulders, arms or upper part of the body, removing superfluous hair, manicuring the nails of any person, *male or female,* and to arrange, dress, curl, wave, cleanse, cut, singe, bleach, color or similarly treat the hair of any *female*." Here also the new profession has not been permitted to infringe upon the immemorial rights of the barber.

Wisconsin found necessity for definitions of the terms bobbing, beauty parlor, managing cosmetician, operator, itinerant cosmetician and school of cosmetic art. It carefully exempts chiropodists, masseurs, hospital attendants, nurses and student nurses, physicians, surgeons and barbers from the operations of the act. It places all cosmetic establishments under the State board of health for examination and inspection. It regulates particularly the use of the electric needle. There must be no treatment of diseases of the skin or scalp except under the direct supervision of a physician. Towels may be used only once and instruments must be sterilized after each employment.

In some of the States the licensing of cosmetic practitioners is controlled by a State board of registration, in some by the board of health, and in some by specially established boards. In New Mexico the board has five members, of whom at least two must be women beauty culturists and two male hairdressers. Nothing is said about the qualifications of the fifth member. Utah mentions specifically as included in the practice of the cosmetician the removing of superfluous hair, warts or moles by the use of electricity or otherwise.

To those familiar with legislative methods in America it will be clear at once that the passage of such legislation in so many States within a period of little more than a year represents an organized movement, with the submission of a so-called model bill, modified to meet the idiosyncrasies of the individual States. "These six laws were obtained," says the official organ of the American Cosmeticians' Society, "as a result of much self-sacrifice and hard work on the part of a small group of women in each of these States. They have behind them some fine organization work, personal enthusiasm that could not be dampened by setbacks and misunderstandings, meetings without number, countless hours of telephoning, hundreds of personal interviews with legislators, weeks given over to lobbying in the State capitals, days of anxiety and disappointment, and a generous amount of that necessary thing—co-operation."

In Missouri success was not difficult because the local branches of the American Cosmeticians' Society and the National Hair-dressers' Association combined forces to push the bill through. But hearken to what happened in Oregon, as told by Miss Mary E. Newman, of the National School of Cosmeticians in Portland:

When the newspapers began to ridicule our movement, many of us who carried the most advertising stopped it immediately, and made a personal appeal to the editors. They reconsidered and gave us a splendid write-up.

We hired no lobbyist—we did our own lobbying. We each tried to look our best and be ladylike, not bold or forward, and we were listened to with respect, though at first there was the usual attitude of ridicule.

Our bill passed through Senate and House by a large majority. But not until the governor had signed our bill did we lessen our vigilance.

The report from New Mexico is almost romantic; thus the leading newspaper of Santa Fé:

When the bill regulating the beauty parlor operators was introduced, great hilarity ensued, and the bill and all its works were greatly kidded. All that was needed for a laugh the first three weeks of the session was a casual reference to the beauty parlor bill. The earnest and good-natured young ladies who lobbied the bill to a triumphant finish dimpled merrily at all the jokes, issued frequent invitations to luncheons and dinners, talked quietly. When the bill came up for passage it was regarded as seriously as any other measure in the House.

Miss Evelyn Lazarus, a worker in the same sovereign State, contributes this record of her personal experience:

Before our bill was presented I had no less than four conferences with the Barbers' Union here in Albuquerque. I can't remember ever having had to do so much fighting before. The argument waxed so hot about what our line of work included that it got into personalities. Then again politics were played. . . .

Then our real trouble was to start—in the House. Over 50 per cent of the House is Spanish, and you just talk at them, not to them. We presented our case to every man there. Every place and any place we met them they were lobbied. [*Sic.*] A few had their wives with them, which was a great help to us.

Miss Pinson has that go-get-it smile, and however discouraged we were, she smiled—in spite of the mean things that were said to us. . . .

What wonder, then, that the passionate legislators of New Mexico succumbed, and made cosmetology a licensed and learned profession!

3

Following the experience acquired by our surgeons in the Great War, plastic surgery advanced very rapidly. The need for restoring extensive segments of the skin, for rebuilding facial contours destroyed by explosives, and for repairing the ravages of burns by fire or chemicals gave birth to surgical methods with results nothing short of marvelous. Such specialists as the English surgeon

Gillies have published vast tomes recording the before and after aspects of hundreds of patients. A dissemination of the photographs marked "before" would make most potent propaganda for the pacifists. But the "after" illustrations, revealing the accomplishments of the surgeons, aided by certain artists in the creation of artificial noses, ears, toupées, and what not, arouse gasps of astonishment and almost of unbelief. However great the skepticism of the reader may be, the facts are nevertheless as depicted by Mr. Gillies.

A few regularly licensed medical men in some of our large cities have built up tremendous practices in such reconstructive surgery. Merely as an estimate, I should guess that there are to-day perhaps ten reputable surgeons in the United States who do any considerable amount of this work. In addition each of our large cities maintains from one to ten practitioners, all regularly licensed but beyond the best repute and wavering on the shadowy borderland of quackery, who likewise limit their practices to facial and body reconstruction. Finally, a considerable number of so-called general surgeons, of surgeons limiting their practice to the ear, nose and throat, and of physicians specializing in diseases of the skin undertake such procedures on occasion.

It is not within the purview of this article to define the marks of the charlatan in plastic surgery. Gradually those marks are becoming apparent even to credulous *Homo americanus*. Some of the "spe-

THE CULT OF BEAUTY 77

cialists" advertise openly in the newspapers, giving
a list of the operations which they wish to undertake. An example follows:

AMERICA'S LEADING
FACE SPECIALIST
AN ETHICAL SURGEON
REGISTERED AND LICENSED
OVER 22 YEARS IN
CHICAGO, ILL.

Many people do not realize that their facial
appearance has so much to do with their success
in business and society. It is true, your personality has much to do with your popularity, but
even with a charming personality the entire
effect is spoiled if you are embarrassed by a
deformed nose of any kind. Sagging Cheeks—
Nose to Mouth Lines, Ruffly-Wrinkly Skin
over and under the Eyes—Scars—Outstanding
Ears—too large or too small a mouth, a loose,
flabby neck or any other deformity or blemish.
For 22 years Dr. —— —— has been a Licensed Surgeon in Chicago, Ill. His knowledge
gained from many years of study and his vast
experience places him in a position to give you
the soundest and most valuable advice just what
can be done in your particular case.

The corrections are done without loss of
time from business or social affairs. No band-
ages are used and all the work is painless.
Phone for appointment. Privacy is assured
you at all times; separate entrance and exit.

The appeal to secrecy is one of the mainstays of
the trade. The successful results are broadcast by

the patient himself and by the charlatan through the press and through his advertising literature, but the patient who has had an unsuccessful result is likely, if he lives, to hide his chagrin in silence. Occasionally, when the results are especially serious, they come to light through the medium of the courts. From several hundreds of instances that are available I select a few:

Los Angeles, Cal.—Suit for $500,000 damages has been filed here against Drs. —— —— and —— ——, plastic surgeons, by Mrs. — — ——. In her complaint, Mrs. —— states the defendants attempted to remove superfluous flesh from her ankles, but that it finally became necessary to amputate both legs.

Chicago.—Dr. —— ——, plastic surgeon, . . . to-day is defendant in a damage suit for $7,000. . . . In her bill Mrs. —— states that as a result of facial treatments a year ago her face was badly scarred and her eyes so badly crossed she was obliged to have them straightened by another surgeon "at great cost and suffering to herself."

Chicago.—Dr. — — —— is the defendant in a suit for $50,000, filed in the Superior Court yesterday. . . . The bill charges that on July 17, Dr. —— performed an operation to straighten ——'s eyes. As a result of carelessness and insanitary conditions under which the operation was performed, according to the bill, ——'s eyes became infected and it was later necessary for another surgeon to remove one of them.

A dignified, handsomely dressed woman walked into my office in Chicago in September, 1926. When she removed her hat and her veil her face revealed the wreckage of an encounter with one of the most widely advertised plastic surgeons in America. She had come to him only after Gillies, some French surgeons and several in New York had told her to avoid plastic surgery. But when she was a girl she had been operated on for removal of some glands in the neck and she considered the scar unsightly when she wore an evening gown.

The Chicago surgeon consented to remove the scar from the neck, inveigled the lady into a face-peeling operation, and undertook to do his surgery in his office under a local anesthetic. The results were pitiful. The caustic acid used in the face peeling had produced scarring worse than the original condition. The original scar had been operated on twice and as sometimes occurs in such cases, the new scars were far worse than the old. Portions of the eyebrows had been removed and the contraction of the scar had left an extremely distorted appearance.

Because of the prominence of her social position the woman could not go into court to seek financial reparations for the injury done to her body. The complaisant medical laws of the State of Illinois make it a haven for all practitioners who can gain a license since this valuable scrap of paper once obtained by hook or crook can be removed only on conviction of a felony.

One plastic surgeon who is reputed to be most successful—only, however, from the point of view of the size of his income—has for several years employed a publicity representative who is charged with the duties of securing patients of note, particularly in the theatrical profession, with the wide dissemination of news of successful results, with the suppression of newspaper statements about unsuccessful results, and with the promotion of publicity concerning unsuccessful surgery by and damage suits against competitors.

In many instances the records of these plastic surgeons are befogged by doubts as to whether or not they have ever had medical or surgical training sufficient to qualify them for undertaking the most simple of operations. Indeed, it is not clear in some cases that they have even graduated from reputable medical schools or obtained their licensure by proper examination. The aspirant for facial reconstruction will do well to inquire carefully into these matters before submitting himself to the scalpel.

The competent performer of plastic surgery gets his results by the transplantation of flaps of tissue from one portion of the body to another. The manipulation is delicate, usually demanding the retention of the original blood-supply of the part until a new blood-supply develops at the spot to which the transfer is made. Obviously here is a procedure to be carried out only in a good hospital and under the most aseptic conditions. The growth of such tissue may require weeks or months. Sometimes a portion of cartilage is transferred also, say to build up the sunken bridge of a nose that gives the face a dished appearance. The procedure of the charlatan is to fill a syringe with melted paraffin and to inject this beneath the skin to fill out the cavity. The paraffin hardens and the patient is satisfied. But experience has shown that paraffin has the peculiar quality of stimulating the growth of the tissue-cells, and numerous cases are now on record of the development of disfiguring tumors and even of cancers after its injection.

On a hot day in July in 1924 there came into my editorial sanctum a young woman accompanied by a somewhat elderly man. "Look at that nose," she said, and with the words demonstrated how the organ referred to might be turned right, left, upward or downward according to the direction in which her fingers impelled it. "Dr. —— did that," she said. "He promised me that he wouldn't use paraffin, and then when he got me in the chair he injected it. We've already paid him $300 for taking the bags out from under Joe's eyes, but this is terrible." And Joe, whose eyes still bagged a little, interjected: "I held the umbrella over her all the way over here so that nose would stay up until we got here." The lady had small chance of redress, for a complaisant State finds it difficult to interfere with the practitioners that it has once licensed, and the charlatans, anticipating difficulties, are protected by insurance companies which agree to fight their damage suits.

An especially rich field for the plastic surgery quack is the child or adult suffering from cross-eye. The majority of the cases are caused by eye-strain accompanying far-sightedness. Nowadays the eyes are first examined by a competent eye specialist and corrective glasses are tried before any operations are attempted. But the plastic surgery quack guarantees to cure by a simple operation, knowing that his guarantee is worthless. In more severe cases due to a deficiency of the muscles of the eye, surgeons who have specialized in the work will shorten a muscle or change its place of insertion. Each case demands careful study and accurate measurements which the plastic surgery quack is not competent to make and he can never obtain a competent eye specialist to help him. In several instances after enough patients have suffered the loss of an eye, State officials have been able to secure cancellation of the license to practice.

Cosmetic operations are most commonly sought by elderly women in love with young men, by aging actresses eager to continue profitably as ingénues, by women whose husbands have lost interest in them, by pugilists who have fought to financial success at the cost of facial continuity, and finally by foolish little salesgirls, stenographers, clerks, aspirants to the movies, sheiks, and what not. The most popular operation, perhaps, is that for the reconstruction of the nose, the most unsatisfactory organ ever devised by an all-wise Creator. The perfect heroine for novelists stands waiting: she is the impossible young woman who is perfectly satisfied with the nose that she was born with. There come then the correction of outstanding ears, the reconstruction of cauliflower or tin ears, the removal of "bags" beneath the eyes, the so-called face-lifting for the elimination of wrinkles or of jowls that have sagged, the excision of double chins, and, finally, the removal of fat, principally from the thighs, the hips, the buttocks, the abdomen and the breasts.

When these operations are performed by competent surgeons under the best of conditions the results are frequently successful—provided, however, (a) that there is no secondary infection, (b) that the tissues of the patient have sufficient recuperative power, (c) that the skin of the patient does not tend to the overgrowth of the scar tissue called "keloid," (d) that the accumulation of fat is not due to some inherent disturbance of the bodily processes particularly involving the glands of internal secretion, and (e) that the surgeon is lucky. Unfortunately, there are records of hundreds of cases in which the surgeons were *not* lucky—indeed,

so many that reputable surgeons hesitate to undertake such procedures unless the defects are fla-
grantly disfiguring or involve a serious disability.
During and after the war the government provided
the wherewithal for stays of many months in hospital for soldiers undergoing repeated reconstructive
operations. In the great manufacturing industries
patients are sometimes severely injured through in-
advertent contact with Frankensteinian machines,
and it becomes necessary to rebuild features or to
replace scalps that have been torn away. Great
hospitals and funds are available for carrying on
such surgical procedures. But only a few really
competent surgeons find time or inclination for the
type of plastic surgery performed wholly for
esthetic reasons. That is the field which has been
invaded and which is largely controlled by
charlatans.

4

Somewhere toward the end of those vaudeville
acts in which a young gentleman and a young lady
indulge in acrimonious remarks relative to the merits
of the sexes, the lady is likely to remark: "Well,
in one way a woman is smarter than a man, any-
how." "What's that?" asks the feeder. "Well, you
take a bald-headed man, he buys hair-tonic; but a
woman buys hair."

The truth in the jest is apparent. The promotion,

retention and replacement of the hirsutage which is
a surviving vestige of *Pithecanthropus erectus* gives
occupation to thousands of men and women. The
changes of fashion in coiffures, the invention of
electrical devices of Goldbergian intricacy for making curls and waves, the creams, lotions, oils and
pastes for washing and giving luster to the hair,
require the services of thousands of experts. The
current styles of bobbing, shingling or otherwise
trimming what used to be called woman's crown-
ing glory have made the barber-shop a delicately
scented boudoir without even a cuspidor. Finally,
there are the diseases of the hair resulting from infection with parasites, bacteria or fungi, which give
concern to the medical specialist in dermatology.
With the desirability or not of the current styles I
am not here concerned, for I am inquiring more particularly into matters of fraud and deceit.

Among all the fallacies attaching to the care of
the hair none is so persistent as the belief in the virtues of the so-called singe, recommended to overcome splitting at the ends and to prevent the falling
out of the hair. The tonsorial artist avers that the
burning of the tip will close the pores and keep the
fluid in the hair. Actually, singeing merely substitutes a charred blunt end of fused horn for one
tapering to a point or cut clean across. In fact,
splitting of the ends is more easily controlled by
greasing the hair lightly and supplying it with the
fat that is lacking. Singeing the hair-ends in order

to prevent the fluid from escaping is based on the misconception that the hair has a central cavity through which it is supplied with some sort of nourishing sap. The hair has no more sap than a buggy-whip; it is nourished only by the blood that reaches its root. Above the surface it is simply a spine of horn, which can be oiled from without.

The removal of superfluous hair is one of the most delicate tasks that can confront the dermatologic specialist. The fact is recognized by those state laws which, as has been mentioned, throw special safeguards around this procedure and define the specialty of "electrologist." Most dermatologists are agreed that the one certain method for permanent depilation is the use of the electric needle. The procedure is time-consuming, somewhat painful, and only from five to twelve hairs are removed in an ordinary treatment. There exist numerous chemical depilatories containing caustic substances, but they irritate the skin at the same time that they remove the hair, and since they do not destroy the hair roots they do not remove the hair permanently. There exists also the possibility of removing superfluous hair by the use of the X-ray. This method is followed by numerous so-called "Tricho Institutes," established throughout the country. But the X-ray is a two-edged sword, possessing great possibility for serious harm, as well as possibility for good when used by those familiar with its dangers. Already specialists in diseases of the skin are reporting the occurrence of hardening of the upper layers of the skin, or overgrowth of the cells, known scientifically as precancerous keratosis, in persons subjected to such treatments. In many of the colleges for the training of those who wish to devote themselves to the beauticians' art attempts are made to instruct in the uses of such apparatus, but the business itself is so new and the teachers themselves, in most instances, are so poorly informed concerning the actual anatomy, physiology and pathology of the skin that it may be said without fear of overstatement that the majority of persons now using these methods are not competent.

The removal of moles, warts and other excrescences upon the skin is another branch of "cosmetology" that presents dangerous possibilities. For years physicians have warned against interference, except by the most careful surgery, with moles of a deeply pigmented character.

Numerous instances are reported in which cutting, burning, or otherwise tampering with such moles has resulted in the appearance of cancerous tumors and their rapid dissemination throughout the body, resulting in death. The ability to distinguish between such defects as are benign and such as are dangerous comes only with extensive study. Obviously, that knowledge is not to be acquired either by a year's apprenticeship in a beauty shop or by six months in a beauty "college."

5

Since the profits of the beauty shop are dependent mainly upon the sale of lotions, creams, shampoos, ointments, depilatories, beauty clays, face packs and similar preparations, the number of these increases daily. Preparations similar to most of the beauty clays, costing at retail from $2 to $10 a pound, may be made by mixing a pound of kaolin, or dried beauty clay, with the same weight of water. Such a preparation costs 20 cents. Nevertheless, pages in most of the periodicals addressed primarily to women contain full page announcements of Terra-derma-lax, Boncilla, Domino Complexion Clay, Mineralava, and Forty-Minute Beauty Clay.

Despite the advertisements, it is quite impossible to feed the skin by rubbing in fats or creams of any kind. Nor is cleanliness aided by plastering the surface of the skin with one type of cream after another and then being compelled to wash away the entire mess. There is no such thing as a skin-food. The skin can be soothed, inflamed, or made temporarily more pliable by external applications, but it cannot be fed. Dozens of preparations for the control of pimples and blackheads are employed by adolescents, both male and female, but genuine specialists in diseases of the skin are likely to recommend simple washing, with the applications of antiseptic solutions that may be purchased for a few cents.

Mixtures to be used in the bath for the reduction of weight commonly consist of baking soda or Epsom salts slightly perfumed, and are sold for twenty to fifty times their original cost. There is, in fact hardly a single possibility in this field that has not been astutely exhausted by the manufacturers of cosmetic nostrums.

Physicians who conduct newspaper columns devoted to answering questions from readers find that at least half of their correspondence is concerned with the problem of entrancing the opposite sex by displays of healthy beauty. Warn as one will of the folly of dependence on the cosmetic nostrum, of its inertness and sophistication, hope springs eternal and the sales go on. There is no limit to the field that the cosmetician approaches. The very acme is reached in the following quotation:

> The warm, pink glow of a perfectly rounded elbow is a joy unconfined to the exacting woman whose social obligations are insistent and many. Harriet I. Nash has made a Perfect Elbow possible to all by her elbow beautifier. The wrinkles and dullness common to many elbows are no longer embarrassments to be endured.

As for the results, one need not have an eye that is unusually discriminating to see that the building up of this vast trade has not resulted, on the whole, in lending a more comely appearance to the current American scene.

CHAPTER III

THE CRAZE FOR REDUCTION

BEFORE modern medical science developed our present knowledge of calories and vitamins, of exercise and massage, of electrical apparatus and thyroid extracts, consideration of the body weight was a relatively simple matter. A woman in those days was either fat or thin, and that was all there was to it. The one successful career that was open to her was a rather permanent marriage. Then, almost overnight, newspapers began to carry the advertisements of nostrums of varying efficiency and danger guaranteed to speed up the body activities and to lessen its absorption of food. Phonograph records and the radio spouted systematic calisthenics or tunes to which women rolled or somersaulted upon the floor. Retired pugilists became the favorite consultants of ladies of leisure and fashion, who embarked determinedly on careers of rope-skipping and weight-lifting. Intricate electrical manipulating, molding or vibrating devices were offered to the susceptible of ample figures and means, and the department stores stocked up on strangely distorted rolling-pins with which milady conceived the fat of the body might be pleasantly distributed less noticeably about the person.

There seems, indeed, to have come upon the women of America a veritable craze for reduction which has passed the bounds of normality and driven women and young girls to a type of self-mutilation impossible to explain on any other basis than the faddism of the mob. How is one to understand the voluntary regurgitation of food after eating, a system commonly used by growing girls in our large cities? The intensive smoking before meals to destroy appetite has become so habitual that men offer the cigarette-case to their dinner partners immediately on becoming seated at the table. Intricate devices for weight reduction form the center of establishments which thrive on the patronage of women.

Of all of the fads that have afflicted mankind none seems more difficult of scientific exposition than the craze for slenderization. Indeed, the only serious explanation that has been offered is that this action represents an attempt of women to adapt themselves to ready-made garments offered in the shops and stores.

It is no new thing to psychologists to see either men or women adapting their bodies to unreasonable fads. There is the compression of the feet by Chinese women, the pressing of the head by the "flat-head" Indians of North America, the mutilation of the nostrils and the ears by the savages of Africa and the overdevelopment of breasts encouraged by the Hottentots. No doubt all of these distortions and mutilations are dangerous from the health point of view, but unquestionably none of them is so serious from this aspect as is the craze for reduction. The unchangeable requirements of nature which associate womanhood with childbirth cannot be gainsaid. Adequate nutrition is absolutely essential to normal childbirth, not only from the point of view of proper nourishment of the infant before birth, but also as it concerns the health of the mother previous to and following birth. True, the presence of excessive fat is a menace in this as in all other physical conditions, but it should be emphasized that the present craze for reduction of the weight to a point involving the removal of even that fatty tissue which constitutes a normal reserve may lead to fatalities under certain conditions. The relationship of undernutrition to anemia, tuberculosis and other wasting diseases is as certainly established as any factor in medicine.

National and racial tastes in the matter of feminine fat and configuration have always varied. The German and the Scandinavian types prefer women comfortably cushioned with body fat, tall, Junoesque and stately. These preferences are reflected in the paintings of their masters in art. The more recent English susceptibility to rather long-limbed, slim-flanked, easy-striding girlish models is emphasized by the description of heroines in English novels of our period. The modern American girl featured on magazine covers and in the rotogravure

sections of the press is a thin, sometimes quite
angular, girl with a posture quite different from that
assumed by the damsel of twenty-five years ago.
Obesity of women is greatly admired among Oriental
races in which the supremacy of man is unchallenged.
Every one recognizes the Turkish predilection for
women comfortably supplied at selected portions of
the anatomy with cushions of adipose tissue. Stratz,
a German ethnologist, has collected photographs
of the typical women of all races. The measurements he records show the hopelessness of attempting to bring all women to one standard of weight,
height, and body form. It must be remembered that
the American woman is, after all, the end product of
a mixture of races. The type, if predominantly
Anglo-Saxon, is nevertheless subject to the modify-
ing influences of European stocks.

Moreover, a certain distribution of the fat beneath the skin is characteristic of the body of all
women. This distribution obviously represents the
attempt of nature to provide for definite feminine
functions. Psychologists are convinced that if these
prerequisites of women are heedlessly ignored,
serious dissociations of the personality may result.
Nevertheless, the craze for thinness has seized upon
womankind like a new catchword or the cross-word
puzzle.

It is rather interesting to speculate as to whether
or not the fad for slenderization is the result of the
rise of feminism and the passing of some eleven mil-

lions of women out of the home and into industries and occupations which were formerly the prerogatives of men. Such modifications as the thinning of the figure, the binding of the breast, the bobbing of the hair and the simplification of the costume may result from a desire for greater ease of movement required by a change in the character of women's work. They are likely, however, to be far more significant, since they involve the removal or suppression of fundamental feminine secondary sex characters. "Care should be taken," warns Dr. Stewart Paton, eminent psychologist, "to distinguish between those women with an intelligent wish to attain political equality and those with ill-defined longings, which are merely the expression of imperfect adjustment."

The students of human behavior point to France as a nation which has been perhaps less prominently identified with efforts to emancipate women than any other of the nations leading in modern civilization. It is significant that French women have not, at least to anywhere nearly the same extent as American women, succumbed to the craze for emaciation. France, has, indeed, given demonstration of the advisability of cultivating manly and womanly qualities without sacrificing the normal feminine traits of character. Psychologists view with alarm the present tendency in this country to underestimate the importance of retaining for women the distinctively feminine traits. Paton considers the modern American young woman subject to an insidiously dangerous form of egotism, which may eventuate in a serious disturbance of the social status of the home in our civilization.

It is rather interesting to speculate also as to whether the change in type of women is the result of the change in dress or vice versa. It seems logical to believe that the changing position of woman in the social scheme conferred upon her duties and opportunities which demanded a change in costume, if not a change in body form. Consider, for example, the dress worn by the woman of 1890 to 1900. The underclothing was abundant, to say the least; the corset was a powerful armor of steel, whalebone, canvas and silk, which was planned to produce a constriction of the waist. There resulted no doubt in many instances a malformation of the body which gave concern to the physicians. The text-books of hygiene of a previous generation had much to say concerning the "corset-liver" and the distorted figure. No wonder that hygienists welcomed the discarding of the corset and development of the modern type of the body support with salvos of applause. Covering the corset were long skirts, full waists, and not infrequently high lace collars, the latter somewhat further bolstered by awkward and irritating celluloid or bone contraptions. What marvel that women celebrated their emancipation from this blanketing with three rousing cheers! The times were ripe for a change in fashion. But the evolution of feminine dress has never been the gradual sort of process that occurs in nature's molding of the human or animal form. It tends rather to sudden and astonishing changes that approach the extreme range of the pendulum.

In the first volume of "Our Times," Mark Sullivan pictures the changing trend of feminine fashions since 1900. In that year a dry-goods salesman, representing one of the nation's largest manufacturers, said: "The shirt-waist has come to stay." Three years later the Chicago *Tribune* heralded its passing with the simple phrase: *"Vale* the shirt-waist." Logical as it may seem to believe that the figure of woman controls the styles and that the necessities of her existence have a definite bearing, a study of the styles seems to lead to the well-established opinion that woman has always somewhat unreasonably adapted her physical body to the styles and permitted the necessities of her existence to make the best of it.

Excess of fat is not due merely to excess of calories taken into the body over the amount used in work. Every one knows that there are persons inordinately thin who eat tremendous amounts of food and who exercise but little. There are, likewise, fat people who eat lightly and exercise much but continue fat. It would be foolish to deny to any woman that she can starve herself thin, or to tell the thin one that she cannot increase her weight by taking an excess of food. Nevertheless, two persons of equal height, fed equal amounts of similar food, may differ enormously, due to internal conditions associated with the disturbances of the glands of internal secretion, with the results of disease or with other undefinable factors. In such instances, attempts to decrease the body weight by starvation, by exercise, by manipulation, by drugs, or by any other well-known methods, are futile.

The argument has been advanced that the modern boyish figure is more beautiful than the curves of an earlier day. Yet it is easy to remember when curves were considered most beautiful. Beauty is in no sense of the word an actual quality of anything, but is wholly of the mind. It is a purely suggestive phenomenon, as is realized when one considers the beautiful according to various racial and national standards. After all, the really beautiful is that which is healthful and efficient, or that which most closely approximates the work of nature. Yet the present craze for thinness is an attempt to modify the processes of nature in a manner against which nature itself seems to revolt.

CHAPTER IV

REJUVENATION

THERE is no fool like an old fool—particularly in matters of rejuvenation. For the senile, tottering old men, leering passion and desire, the world has only the pity that it confers on a Faust, who bartered his soul for a few years of youthfulness; the ridicule that it darts upon a Don Quixote; the mild amusement with which it listens to the tale of Ponce de Leon; or the savagery with which it attacks the decrepit prey of physical lusts inspired by inflamed tissues, who slakes his inordinate appetites with the inveiglement of young girls. Behind all of these legends and observations lie the insights of historians who have seen fundamental biologic instincts expressing unsatisfied and hopeless desires. Here psychologists observe the last expression of the law of self-preservation, the reaction of the living toward approaching death, the feeble call on unresponsive nerves and muscles for power that they cannot give. To-day the public is told again and again in sensation-mongering newspapers and periodicals that the secret of restoring youthful vigor to worn out tissues has been solved in the laboratories of the Austrian Steinach and of the

Frenchman Voronoff. Alas! medical scientists who like to be shown before they are convinced, mistrust the evidence. They grant readily that the senescent graybeard with the will-to-believe may be instilled with young ideas, but they have yet to admit that any surgical operation, any transplantation of glands, any decoction of plant, organ or mineral remedies will confer on the withered form the machinery to put those ideas into action. Of the mechanical contrivances, the glandular extracts, and the other forms of hocus-pocus sold with claims for their ability to rejuvenate more will be said in the next chapter. Now and here the disciples of the scalpel who are reaping somewhat of a harvest in the field of surgical rejuvenation will receive our discriminating, if not too tender attention.

Man's search for the elixir of eternal youth was never a scientific one previous to the period of Brown-Sequard. Long before Brown-Sequard, however, anatomists and physiologists had been studying the nature and the functions of the male sex glands. It had been shown that the ability to reproduce was coördinate with certain changes in the body of the child that are known as the secondary sex characters. The voice of the boy deepens, causing great embarrassment when a fine soprano statement suddenly changes to a basso growl. The first inklings of mustache and beard send him to his mirror for hours of painstaking scrutiny. He begins to take a more serious interest in the female of the species.

And it was taken for granted that the development of these sex characters was the result of a special or internal secretion poured into the blood by the sex glands. In science, however, it is not well to take anything for granted.

In 1889, the famous French physiologist thought that he had discovered the potent substance in the extracts of male sex glands. One need not be a Freudian to realize that the terms vim, vigor, virility or vitality are almost invariably associated with sexual power and the ability to engage in the act of reproduction. It was not strange, therefore, that attention should be turned to these organs in the search for the important substance. Indeed, the most primitive savages of cannibalistic nature were wont themselves to brew essences of the organs of the enemies whom they slew in battle, believing that the ingestion of the tissues was sufficient to confer upon them the prowess of their vanquished foes. Nor is it surprising that Brown-Sequard, having inoculated himself with extracts of sex organs developed a sort of similitude of youthfulness. He reported that he could now climb a flight of steps with greater rapidity and ease than before his inoculation. Nevertheless, at the appointed time, the body of Brown-Sequard went the way of all flesh. And the skeptical scientists who repeated his experiments, checking them with numerous cases and controlling them with injections of plain water instead of the extracts, shook their heads in dismay. The great scientist—for Brown-Sequard was all of that —had yielded science to enthusiasm and his conclusions could not be sustained.

THE THEORY OF STEINACH

The conception on which the Steinach operation for rejuvenation is based, the delicate details of the operation, will require perhaps somewhat too much of delicacy in their description for easy comprehension.

About 1903 two French biologists claimed that the secretion responsible for maleness was developed by a certain part of the male sex gland. They asserted that this portion of the gland developed particularly if the tubes leading from the gland were tied off so that the portion responsible for producing the male cells of reproduction would degenerate. And Steinach claimed that he had confirmed their experiments and that the performance of this operation on senescent animals resulted in rejuvenation.

Now the finding of a substance or a system of rejuvenation is much like the finding of gold. Whether it is there or not, all of the unsuccessful, romantic, and adventurous experimenters rush in on the trail, and all of the aged and worn out capitalists come in as soon as convenient to take advantage of the discovery. The cry of "gold, gold" was taken up quickly by a number of young and enthusiastic investigators, who followed Steinach. Some famous actors, physicians, and financiers who saw the waning

of their power and note and of their ability to enjoy
to the utmost the lives that had given them so much
became subjects of the experiment. Where there
are actors, authors and financiers, there is also always in these modern times, good newspaper publicity. And where there is newspaper publicity not
too careful as to the facts, there are soon more ap-
plicants for operations. This, in medical science,
is known as a vicious circle.

The careful experimenters who have followed the
work of Steinach, checking all his results carefully
on experimental animals, have demolished his claims
bit by bit. Oslund of the Vanderbilt Medical School
showed that the Steinach adherents had been de-
ceived because of the type of experimental animal
used. Since the theory of rejuvenescence is based
on an overdevelopment of the cells within the sex
gland that does not actually occur, it can be taken
for granted that cutting of the ducts with the idea
of producing such overdevelopment cannot cause
rejuvenescence. And the work of Oslund has been
confirmed by Moore and many others.

In a recent consideration of the topic of rejuvenation, Dr. William T. Belfield demolishes the belief
that the sex glands are responsible for the development of the secondary sex character in two succinct
statements: The complete sex features of mind and
body, including the external sex organs, have been
found in persons in whom the so-called sex glands
were absent from birth, as proved by complete post-

mortem examination. Furthermore, all of the sex features of the male sex, including the external organs, have been found in persons in whom the sex glands were absent from birth, but who had within the body a complete set of female sex glands. There is a great deal of much more technical evidence to support the view that the sex glands are not the only tissues concerned with establishing maleness or femaleness of any individual. Perhaps the best of it developed in experiments on hens and roosters, revealing hens possessing the comb and wattles and even the feathers of the rooster, yet living a hen's life, laying eggs and hatching them out! But what, you ask, has all of this to do with Steinach's theory of rejuvenation?

The elderly gentleman who prefers blondes is hardly likely to be deterred, by the details of technical experiments on mice, rabbits, chickens or dogs. For him, therefore, one presents the facts regarding man. For many years the operation now called the Steinach rejuvenation operation was performed on old men who suffered from enlargement of another organ closely associated with the sexual tissues. This gland—the prostate—first received newspaper respectability when its enlargement in the case of a noted holder of public office gave it great diplomatic importance. But in not one of the hundreds of cases of cutting of the ducts reported previous to the time of Steinach did any of the meticulous surgeons who reported the cases mention any restoration of youthful vigor or anything resembling rejuvenation. This fact has been called to the attention of Steinach and of all his followers again and again in reputable medical publications.

To the proof of the scientific laboratory investigators that the Steinach method is founded on fallacy, the Steinach adherents and the surgeons who perform the Steinach operation reply with the sort of cynical shrug of the shoulders that such practical men use in answering laboratory evidence. They point with none too reluctant pride to their records of cases operated on and to the letters of testimony. Here is as simple a gesture as might be made by a moron, but hardly the sort of thing one expects from a scientist. The same testimonials—in fact much stronger ones—can be found for all of the nostrums and contrivances that have invaded this fertile field.

Opposed to the enthusiastic statement of Adolph Lorenz, to whom personal newspaper exploitation is no novelty, is that of Professor M. Zeissl of Vienna, that the only change he noted after his operation was less frequent sex desire than previously. Opposed to the insidious publicity of Dr. Harry Benjamin of New York concerning the one hundred cases on which he operated with a claimed considerable percentage of success are the records hidden away in medical literature of thousands and thousands of men on whom such operations were done without any noticeable response.

There are, indeed, some records of senile men who

put upon their degenerated tissues far more of stress than they could tolerate. Here the illusion of vigor produced an earlier death than might reasonably have occurred without the operation and in the absence of illusion. It is in connection with this phase of the matter that the feline comes leaping forth from the enveloping sack in which it has heretofore been somewhat cautiously concealed.

The prime exponent of the Steinachian miracle in this land that so readily accepts overnight miracles seems to be the aforementioned Dr. Harry Benjamin. In the earlier publications of this disciple one finds no mention of any possible mental effects associated with the surgical procedure. But quite recently, regardless of the fact that this medico is without status in the field of psychology and psychiatry, he begins to mutter somewhat vaguely concerning the importance of coincident psychoanalysis. And in the publicity concerning his efforts appearing within the past two months appears what is, for so shrewd a man, a most incautious admission: "The experts declare that the value of the Steinach method has been much reduced by ignorance and by the opposition of doctors who have mistaken ideas regarding the operation." In other words, the patient must believe thoroughly that the operation will give him vim, vigor and vitality, or he doesn't get it. For many years, physicians who have specialized in the diseases of the sex organs have emphasized again and again the great part played by the mind in controlling their functions. The records of the surgeons who do the Steinach operations are without scientific controls. To what extent have they checked their work by cases on whom the operation was not done, but who otherwise were put through the same procedure? Obviously such controlling of cases would be a most elementary and simple procedure, but records of such control in the publications of the promoters are sadly lacking.

Indeed, these exponents of surgical art would seem to be providing for the future in their claim that the operation may be repeated with good effect and a second revival of powers bestowed on the waning patient. Here is a biologic revolution that bewilders the imagination! The young men, handicapped in competition because of lack of experience and of the world's goods, will be compelled to struggle against their rejuvenated fathers and grandfathers, while the latter, by repeated operations, maintain a permanent lead. It's a sad, sad outlook; but fortunately it isn't true.

The Voronoff Conception

The contention of Voronoff, like that of Steinach, has to do with the use of sex gland material for purposes of rejuvenation. He does not, however, depend on any change in the tissues brought about by tying off ducts. He actually transplants the entire glands, and since the human material is not easily and generally available, attempts to supply the deficiency with glands derived from the anthropoid apes. In this instance also a vast amount of experimental evidence from the past and from other workers of the present is available to disprove the contention that either virility or vigor depend primarily on secretion from the sex glands. True, there are instances in which there is obvious deficiency of the sex glands and in which the transplantation of such material results in conserving useful existence, but the records again are not such as will convince any scientific reader of the merit of the operation. In the first place there is not in any sense of the word actual prolongation of life, since none of those on whom the transplants have been done seem to live beyond the normal period. In the second place, one reads such conclusions as the following: "The pessimistic attitude of the patient and constant brooding over his inability have marred the results of the treatment." Here again the part played by the will-to-believe seems paramount. When all of the evidence is assembled and considered *en masse,* it becomes apparent that there is not as yet any actual proof that rejuvenation has been accomplished in a single individual, or any basis for the belief that it ever will be accomplished. There is, on the other hand, much evidence that a few surgeons, whose names are seen more often in the newspapers than in scientific periodicals, have found rejuvenation operations most valuable in their practice. Valuable to whom?

CHAPTER V

REJUVENATION: THE MECHANICAL AND GLANDULAR METHODS

REJUVENATION is, in these days of young old-men and old young-men, a word to conjure with. The astute purveyors of mechanical devices, pills, lotions and systems of physical culture sold by the mail-order plan have been quick to realize the wonderful "come-on" possibilities inherent in the word. The result has been the interminable repetition of the claim for renewed youth achieved through hundreds of substances and appliances. The post office department itself is hardly able to keep pace with the new developments in the field and its fraud orders are issued usually after the promoters have reaped a fine harvest.

MECHANICAL REJUVENATION

The senescent man or the youthful individual who finds himself suddenly lacking in sexual vigor is a ready prey for the exploiters of mechanical devices which are urged because of their ability to encourage a physical development that seems to be lacking. The average man in this land of unenlightenment regarding his physical constitution has but slight conception of what constitutes the normal in these affairs, either as to physical development or functional ability. Indeed, the more he meditates upon the matter, the more he is likely to be convinced that he himself is sadly lacking in these particulars, the psychology of this view being dependent upon a will to achieve rather than on actual knowledge. Moreover, the cleverly worded literature—and what a sad use of the word this is—of the salesman of various devices is calculated to intensify and emphasize this view. All of the advertising matter is a pæan of praise of sexual athleticism, and a weeping and wailing, inspired to make still more mournful the sexually despondent male.

On December 5, 1925, the post office department issued a fraud order against the manufacturers of a device known as the "Perfection Developer," one Walter H. Hartman of Columbus, Ohio, selling under the firm name of "Hart & Co." The simple device was merely a cylinder of glass connected with a pump and designed to induce a vacuum about the organs to be developed. The effects persisted only so long as the device was in actual use, and if it had any permanent effects whatever, they could only be for harm.

Another device of the same type was sold by one M. Von Schwartz and William Billings of Ithaca, New York, under the name of the "Burt Vacuum Tube." This firm was debarred from the mails September 1, 1925.

These devices are typical of most of the mechanical appliances offered by mail for men lacking sexual vigor. Obviously, they can be of no permanent service. Moreover, the psychology of their use is such as to discourage any real possibility of improvement through rest, diet and psychotherapy which long experience has shown are of value.

GLANDULAR REJUVENATORS

Public interest in any new medical development is at once capitalized by the promoters of nostrums and fallacies. It is not surprising, therefore, that increasing interest and knowledge of the glands of internal secretion should have aroused in the minds of some promoters the possibility of unusual and unwarranted gains.

In March, 1921, the "Youth Gland Chemical Laboratories" was incorporated in Illinois; in February, 1922, the name of the corporation was changed to the "Druesen-Kraft Chemical Laboratories." Later, it became known as the "Lewis Laboratories." It was not, however, until March 19, 1925, that the United States Government closed the mails to this concern. In the meantime, it reaped a rich harvest from the unwary. The advertising literature of this concern was of a style so striking as to have merited some better use. A full-page announcement in the newspapers was headed, in two inch high, black type, "YOUR GLANDS WEAR

OUT"; in the center of the page, he-men and she-women danced the one step in close embrace. And here are the phrases that brought the replies:

It is based entirely on the principle of Feeding Actual Gland Substance Direct to the Glands thereby renewing and rejuvenating them.

This method of giving new life to the glands is advocated and endorsed by the leading students of gland therapy throughout the world —including Dr. Arnold Lorand who is generally conceded to be the greatest living authority on this subject.

The actual method of Treatment used by us is the result of exhaustive experiments covering several thousand cases, during the past two years.

The "Lewis" Treatment Is Practically Never Failing.

If You Could Prevent the Wear and Tear on Your Glands Caused by Sickness, Age, Disease, etc., You Would Look and Feel as Young at 70 as at 25. Science However Has Solved the Secrets of the Glands and Now for the First Time Shows You the True Way to KEEP or REGAIN Your Vigor by Feeding and Replenishing the Most Important Glands!

Build Up Your Glands and You Build Up Your Strength and Endurance.

The evidence is clear that the firm did exceedingly well from a financial point of view. The original price of the treatment was $10.00, which, on occasion, could be reduced to $7.50, and, if the victim still failed to succumb, to a special offer of $2.95. The court records in the case showed that the firm had spent at least $300,000.00 in advertising, and that it had a gross annual income of between $250,000.00 and $300,000.00. Nevertheless, scientific evidence has shown that extracts or other preparations of the sex glands are without any power whatever when taken by mouth. They not only fail to produce rejuvenation of the entire body, but even to stimulate to any extent the particular portions of the body in which the applicant for rejuvenation seems to be especially interested.

Another concern, with headquarters in Denver, issued a booklet entitled "The Secret of Staying Young." Here were the testimonials of elderly men, 82, 83 and 84 years of age, who announced that they had lasting benefits from the treatments offered. These testimonials are just as vociferous and emphatic as those of aspirants for youth operated on by the disciples of Steinach. The treatments consisted of nothing more than dried animal glands, taken by mouth, which, as has been said, could not possibly have the effects claimed for them. The concern exploiting these desiccated glands, the "Vital-O-Gland Company," not content with depending on the mental responses of those who took its preparations by mouth, sold at the same time the usual vacuum developer, a glass tube attached to a bicycle pump. When the Government investigated this concern, it found twenty-two girls and five men occupied in sending out the literature. The evidence revealed that the gross income of the concern for 1923 was $176,406.82. Rejuvenation pays!

The Vital-O-Gland Company and the Lewis Laboratories have been barred by the Government from the use of mails, but there still remain many concerns offering, both to physicians and to the public, glandular preparations for rejuvenation or for sexual stimulation. There will always be senescent, somewhat lewd, and sad, old men to waste the funds of their declining years on such powerless pills. The memories of youth become more and more resplendent with the passing years.

The Glandine Laboratories of Chicago and Los Angeles issues a circular with the question "Must We Grow Old?" and with the answer, "Science Says, No." The treatments consist of extracts of the sex glands to be taken by mouth. The Glandex Company of New York advertised in the public press a combination of gland extracts with iron. The International Research Laboratories of Chicago advertised "Baker's Glandol," with a salacious pamphlet emphasizing the rejuvenation of man, and with such headings as "The Most Interesting Thing Is Love. Don't Waste Life. Luck from Boldness and Suppressed Desires." Where is the man who could resist the plea?

The Puritan Laboratories of Nashville, Tennessee, issues "Glandtone," offered with the claim that it will restore youthful vigor to those passing with age. The Walton Chemical Company of Chicago emphasizes the glands and says that a combination of the sex glands, the thyroid, prostate, pituitary and adrenal, hermetically sealed, will defer old age and renew vitality. What of the impudence and psychological cleverness of its warning:

WARNING!

The country is being flooded with literature from so-called "Laboratories," offering to restore Sex STRENGTH in the forms of unsealed "Gland Tablets" or "Liquids."

Such preparations may contain some gland substance, but unless the ingredients are SEALED to preserve their strength, the potency may be entirely gone in a few days.

The Walton Treatment I N S U R E S the STRENGTH of the INGREDIENTS and thousands have found this method SUCCESSFUL even after years and years of previous failure with other methods of treatment.

In fact, fully three out of four who write of their remarkable results with this new method, say they had taken many other Treatments or methods without relief.

Bear in mind that there is not an iota of evidence to show that any preparation of sex glands, singly or in combination, has ever been shown to have the slightest effect on the human body when given by mouth. It was the hope and the belief of Brown-Sequard that he had found such a substance. Even he thought that the taking of sex glands brought about in him a sort of rejuvenation. Yet in the more than fifty years since his passing, and since his claims were disproved, the public has not learned the truth.

RADIUM AND LIGHT

With the coming of the newer discoveries in medicine as to the effects on the human body of radium, the X-ray and ultraviolet light, the agile-minded exploiters of the public's interest in keeping young were again quick to respond with the preparation and sale of such apparatus and material for purposes of rejuvenation. Of course, rejuvenation is not a physical state that can be easily determined accurately. The old man with declining powers is ready to welcome the slightest sign of increasing ability in physical work or in sexual power. He forgets to reason that the rest and the mental stimulation associated with any new method of treatment are likely to bring about the illusion of strength.

The manufacturer of a cabinet lined with incandescent lamps, for example, is not content to claim for it the simple uses of a sweat bath, or of heat produced by incandescent lamps. Ah! No! This simple cabinet becomes as by the wave of a magician's wand, an "Inductive Metabolizing method." And the manufacturer says:

The —— Inductive Metabolizing method gives to the world one of the greatest, if not the greatest, means of rejuvenation of the human organism known to medicine, but the part that is most interesting about this modality is that of its synergetic action with all the recognized methods of rejuvenation now in use—such as gland therapy, radioactive drinking water, baths, etc., as the results obtained by their use, when accompanied by the Inductive Metabolizing treatments, are increased tenfold.

One can almost picture him rubbing his hands in glee as he murmurs: "Rejuvenation: That's the word that gets 'em!"

The makers of apparatus containing radium or the blenders of waters which have been submitted to the rays of this wondrous element urge also its potency for rejuvenation. They point knowingly to the radioactive springs of Germany and Switzerland and cite the records of the old men who have visited those springs and returned home younger in body, if not in years. But they, too, neglect the effects of weeks of rest and freedom from care, of good diet and salubrious surroundings, and possibly—in fact, probably—of enforced inactivity for those portions of the anatomy whose physical functioning persists in remaining the center of interest when rejuvenation is discussed.

"THE NEW SCIENCE OF RADIENDOCRINOLOGY"

If radiation rejuvenates—although of course it doesn't—and if glands rejuvenate—and it has been shown that they do not—then, say the manufacturers of the Radiendocrinator, the combination will get the result. Merely ray the glands with the Radiendocrinator—price $150—and you are there! The booklets are a hodge-podge of exaggerations, fallacies, and confusions regarding chemistry, physics, biology, glands, radium, and what not. But the convincing document is a blue-colored bonded guarantee of satisfaction or money refunded. Couched in language that seems to make the chance of financial loss to the unwary impossible, the guarantee is nevertheless a snare and a delusion. Launched originally by Dr. Herman H. Rubin, New York, as a device to be worn at night over the glands and selling at $1000, the apparatus is now a reflector on a stand and can be purchased for $150. But for pure romance the literature is at least ten times as fanciful.

THE HOPE FOR THE FUTURE

Even the Greek philosophers murmured that physical powers in matters of sex did not always parallel brain capacity. Strange that the sex instinct should be so deeply rooted and so prominent in life that two thousand years of experience has failed to convince men of the truthfulness of that statement.

Modern science has shown the early detection of signs of disease by physical examination, and the establishment of a proper régime of life, including adequate rest, diet, exercise, simple personal hygiene, and freedom from worry will greatly extend the life of the average man. He may quite reasonably hope to live to seventy years and if he is at all careful considerably beyond that age. It behooves him then to grow old gracefully, remembering that much of the greatest work of this world that has been done in art, letters, invention, finance and statesmanship has been done by men well beyond sixty years of age. Their minds were perhaps little given to the purely pleasurable functions of the bodies which constituted the abode for their restless spirits.

CHAPTER VI

BREAD AND SOME DIETARY FADS

THE romance of bread is a story that has been related many times in folk-lore and in written history. The rhapsodist tells of the farmer going forth at dawn to sow the seed. Below the soil the kernel gathers nourishment to reproduce itself a thousand fold. The wheat lifts its stalk to the life-giving sun and rain. Men and the machines assemble for the harvest. Transportation engineers arrange for conveyance of the seed to the mill and carry the flour across the world. The housewife in Scotland turns out her scones; in France, one sees the long loaves of French bread; in Austria, the Vienna loaf; in Poland, the twist, and in our own country, the bread "untouched by human hands." Time and again the epic of the wheat and of the soil—for the epic of the soil is always the story of wheat—has been the theme of novels such as Zola's "Mother Earth," of Knut Hamsun's "Growth of the Soil," of Reymont's "The Peasants," of Herbert Quick's magnificent trilogy of Iowa and the Vandermark family, and of the great story of Frank Norris, "The Pit." The story of bread carries one back constantly to the beginnings of things. In preparing the English system of weights and measures the pennyweight was represented by thirty-two grains of wheat. Indeed, so fundamental was bread to life that the term baker's dozen arose because of the strict laws laid upon bakers in the giving of proper weight, so that the careful and law-abiding members of the trade threw in an extra loaf to assure the customer that he was receiving adequate measure.

Now there was a time when a loaf of bread in these United States was just about as standard an item as a cubist painting. In those days a loaf of bread looked like bread and perhaps served its purpose satisfactorily as a vehicle for butter or jam, but so far as its content, its texture, and its digestibility were concerned, it was best expressed by the letter "X," representing the unknown quantity. Indeed, young ladies became especially famed for their ability to turn out a specimen that would receive the approbation of the community and many a damsel hung a blue ribbon received at the county fair as exhibit A in the parlor to attract prospective marital candidates in her direction. Many a pseudo-humorist waxed wealthy on the jokes he made concerning the product turned out by newly-weds. And since those were the days before beauty shops were as plentiful as candy stores, many a young lady lacking comeliness qualified for the marriage route by her culinary capacity, with special emphasis on what she could do with flour rather than with powder. Those days, fortunately, are gone forever. To-day a loaf of bread is as standard an item as the money that purchases it; the money must look and feel and weigh the same piece for piece; its ingredients must be always the same, and it must yield a certain definite value; in the same way the loaf of bread must have a definite weight, appearance, texture and taste, and must yield a definite food and body building value. To the physician who has to count on bread as an article in the diet of sick and well, it means much to know that there is a standard.

THE VALUE OF FOOD

The scientific study of food has followed certain definite trends. As early as 1840 it was recognized that proteins, fats, carbohydrates, mineral matter and water were the components of food tissues. Continuously thereafter chemists were investigating constituents of food substances, and by 1895 Atwater and his associates in this country had examined and listed the chemical composition of most common foods. About this time also it became common to classify food substances wholly by their caloric value or the amount of energy that they would yield to the body when taken in and properly digested. The next two decades added to this fundamental knowledge observations concerning those mysterious substances known as the vitamins, so that McCollum and Davis were able in 1915 to formulate a theory of adequate diet. At that time they said that a diet must contain in addition to proteins, carbohydrates and fats for energy, inorganic salts for the building of the body and vitamins A and B necessary for proper growth and development. Later additional vitamins became known, so that the alphabetical category includes A, B, C and D quite definitely established, and possibly vitamin X or E necessary for reproduction. When considering the value of any food to-day we take into account all of these various factors, and, as is obvious to almost any one with a fundamental knowledge of foods, no single substance provides all of the necessary elements for adequate nutrition. Milk is, no doubt, the most satisfactory single article of food consumed by man, but even milk is not a complete food when taken over a long period of time as the sole source of nutriment. One of the troubles with milk is that too much bulk is required to satisfy the body's needs. It contains 87 per cent. of water and 13 per cent. of dissolved substances; it happens to be rich in both calcium and phosphorus, whereas many vegetable foods are rather poor in these elements. Indeed, only the milk of animals and the leafy vegetables contain enough calcium to satisfy the needs of man. The element calcium is a most important substance, for the human body is sensitive to changes in the amount of calcium in the circulating blood. Quite recently Collip, co-worker with Banting in the discovery of insulin, has found that the amount of calcium in the blood may be controlled by an extract made from the parathyroid glands, which lie behind the thyroid gland in the throat. Experimenting with this substance he has been able to produce remarkable changes in the body activity, merely by lowering or increasing the amount of calcium in the blood. Milk supplies not only calcium, but also certain proteins, fats and vitamins.

Wheat, and indeed all the cereal grains, seed substances, potatoes, roots and muscle meats lack the constituents that are supplied by milk and the leafy vegetables. The human being is supposed to be intelligent. It has been alleged that the large majority of us are morons and our dietary habits may be taken as evidence for the allegation. A moron, I may add, lest you take the newspaper definition, is an adult whose intellectual development stopped at the age of twelve. There is no law of man or of nature that compels the thinking human being to limit himself to milk, wheat, oranges, nuts or anything else in the food category. If he is really intelligent he will want to make up his diet of a sufficient variety of foods to provide everything necessary for the proper development and stability of his tissues. He will want to satisfy the esthetics of his appetite and the limitations of his digestive apparatus. Investigations have shown that fresh fruits and certain raw vegetables ought to be included in the diet to provide adequate amounts of vitamin C. Scientific studies have shown that the proteins of the muscle of the liver and kidney are more valuable as a supplement to cereals and fats than are the proteins of milk. Indeed, it is not even certain that milk provides an adequate amount of vitamin B, and it is known that various samples of milk differ as to their quantities of vitamins A and C. Eggs contain everything necessary for the growth and maintenance of the body but are poor in calcium and unbalanced in other food principles. On the other hand, oysters, clams and crabs contain all of the uncharacterized food substances, including iodin and vitamin C. The fact that vitamin D is present in fish oil suggests an importance for fish in the diet that has not been previously thought of. Vitamin D, it must be remembered, is a help to proper reproduction and to the avoidance of sterility. Finally, all of the natural, primary food substances, such as milk, butter, fish and what not are not themselves standardized, but vary according to their place of production and their environment previous to use. This hasty review of the elemental values of some of the well-known food substances is indicative of the importance of a varied diet for man. Let us see how bread, as one of the fundamental and staple substances of human diet, has been gradually modified through scientific education and control to develop as nearly as possible a standard, highly nutritious and body building substance.

The Value of Bread

As was intimated in opening this discussion, the bread of the past epoch had no definite constituents.

It was made in many instances from flour, salt, yeast and water alone. In other instances, it was made of the whole wheat and there were, of course, such modifications as bread made with rye, bread made with bran, bread made with raisins and other added constituents. The baker, from the mechanical point of view alone, is not particularly desirous of preparing any special form of bread. He likes to give his customers what they want, and perhaps to approach as nearly as possible what dietary experts think they ought to have. No doubt, like all other business men, he wants to deal in a staple product and not be subject to extensive losses by the sudden growth of elemental and unjustifiable fads. It was, no doubt, with this desire in mind that the bakers' organization established its Institute of Baking, and it was, no doubt, the same principle that urged many bakers of large interests to establish their own chemical laboratories for the study and standardization of their products. The result has been an application of the scientific facts that have been learned relative to diet to modern bread. This application caused the supplementing with milk of the bread made from white flour, salt, yeast and water. The addition of milk directly to the bread rather than dependence on the housewife to give the milk to the family at the table is well warranted, because economical and scientifically satisfactory. This does not mean to say, however, that the milk added to bread is sufficient for all dietary needs; it merely means that a bread made with milk is a better and richer bread than one made without it. In the same way a bread made with raisins or other fruits provides the added constituents of those fruits. All breads furnish energy according to their composition. Modern bread having a scientifically established composition is a sensible food. It contains about 45 per cent. starch and 50 per cent. total carbohydrates and its protein content averages between 9 and 10 per cent. It provides limited amounts of mineral salts, of fats and of the vitamins, but it should be remembered that wheat products provide 42 per cent. of the carbohydrate consumption of the United States and 26 per cent. of the total calories consumed in all food substances. As may well be imagined, a loaf of bread may vary greatly according to the quantity and the nature of the constituents that go into it. A bread made with white flour, yeast, salt, malt extract, sugar, shortening and water will not have the food value of a bread made of the same constituents with the addition of the amount of milk required by modern baking standards. Our Government permits the title, "Milk Bread," if one-third of the liquid used in making the bread is milk. A bread made with five pounds of sweetened, condensed milk per cental of flour contains about one and a half ounces of milk to a pound of bread. Bread may be made of whole wheat and other elements of roughage and of vitamin supply that are lacking in bread made from white flour, and it is possible to prepare bread with wheat germ added to such an extent as to provide twelve times the amount of wheat germ contained in whole wheat bread. But such breads are open to certain objections so far as texture and keeping qualities are concerned. The physician who is prescribing bread as a part of the patient's diet must know the constituents and character of the bread that he prescribes. Indeed, the situation to-day resembles closely the situation that existed in the drug industry before the American Medical Association appointed its Council on Pharmacy and Chemistry, and before the Food and Drugs Act of a little more than a decade past helped to clarify the situation. To-day through the Council on Pharmacy and Chemistry, physicians are provided each year with a book known as "New and Nonofficial Remedies," which gives the analyses, actions and uses of all of the unofficial drug products available to the medical profession. At the same time the Council regularly issues reports concerning such products as are of indefinite composition or for which claims may be made that are not warranted by the actual constituents of the drug preparations. The variety of products offered from time to time by baking organizations that seem to be more concerned with profits than with public health offers opportunity for similar work in the baking industry to keep both the baker and the public informed of the actual basis on which exploiting of nostrum-like products is based. The Institute of Baking has done, and is doing, much in this direction.

BREAD FOR REDUCING

Not long since a baking organization issued, with extensive claims, a bread which bore the slogan "The Enemy of Fat." Letters at once began to come to the American Medical Association headquarters requesting information concerning this product and its actual importance as a part of the diet of those desiring to reduce. In attempting to reply to these questions, *The Journal of the American Medical Association* sought information from the American Institute of Baking and from the Westfield Testing and Research Laboratories. The information revealed that the bread advertised as an "Enemy of Fat" contained from 29 to 33 per cent. of starch and a total carbohydrate content of from 36 to 40 per cent., whereas ordinary bread contained only some 45 per cent. of starch and 50 per cent. of total carbohydrates. Moreover, the bread for the fat contained 18 per cent. of protein as compared with 9 and 10 per cent. in ordinary bread. Clearly from these analyses the bread mentioned had no special value in a diet for those desiring to reduce. Any woman who would eat a smaller amount of ordinary white bread or the same amount of ordinary whole wheat bread and who would follow the rigid diet recommended in each package of the bread with special claims as to value in obesity would be able to reduce just as rapidly and at less expense. These observations caused the Institute of Baking to make the statement that the claims made for weight-reducing breads were misleading and exaggerated. *The Journal of the American Medical Association* supported the Baking Institute with all its force of influence and publicity in its exposure of this quackery. Length of life and fat. Pigs would live longer if they didn't make hogs of themselves.

THE ALL OR NOTHING POLICY

The tendency to attach undue virtues or evils to single factors in the diet has been responsible for much fallacious teaching in public health. Of all of the faddists that occupy the medical scene the food faddists are, no doubt, most eccentric. The vegetarians, who attach undue evils to the eating of meat, base their conclusions on the fact that the anthropoid apes live on nuts, fruits and cereals. The same faddists are likely, nevertheless, to deprecate the facts supporting the theory of evolution and if they do not, "How," asks McCollum, "do they explain the meat diet of the caveman?" The same faddists cite the fact that animals living on a vegetable diet are strong and tractable, while carnivorous animals are ferocious. Who, however, would care to support the contention that the mind of man is governed by the chemical nature of what he eats? It

has been known for years that the sufferer from in-
digestion and the man irritated by chronic attacks
of gall-bladder inflammation or appendicitis is likely
to be irritable, cynical and a generally unsatisfactory
cuss, but it has also been known that many of our
greatest humorists and many of our finest leaders
have been men who abused tobacco and alcohol and
who gorged themselves with food. There is something more to temperament than the eating of steak
or oats. All the old aphorisms such as, "Tell me
what you eat and I will tell you what you are," were
based more on superstition than on the science of
nutrition. Actually there is no conclusive evidence
to support any view as to the dangers of eating
wholesome quantities of any single article of diet,
such as meat, bread, wheat, or any other of the
fundamental substances. However, it is quite
customary for the faddists to concentrate their attention on the exploitation or condemnation of some
single substance. One of the chief shuttlecocks with
which they have amused themselves is the controversy as to the value of white flour as contrasted with
whole wheat flour bread.

WHOLE WHEAT

The very fact that wheat and bread are fundamental substances in the diet of man has made the
exploitation of cereal products and of bread an
attractive field for the exploiter. This, too, has

influenced the manufacture of numerous whole wheat products, for which claims are made that go far beyond the scientific fact.   Indeed, the false and fulsome advertising has been so po ent that even a circular just issued by the Children's Bureau of the United States Government advises the pregnant woman and the nursing mother to limit their diet of bread and cereals to whole grain because of the high mineral and vitamin content.

Let us consider first the manner in which it has been endeavored to relate the consumption of white flour to the cause of cancer.   It is a significant observation in medical history that the advancing of numerous and peculiar theories is a good indication of the lack of any accurate knowledge as to the cause of disease, just as a multiplicity of methods of treatment is a reflection of a similar state of affairs.   Fortunately sufficient is known about cancer to warrant the advice that it be treated primarily by early diagnosis and surgical removal, with possible application of radium or X-ray for such purposes as may be accomplished with these methods. The world was surprised not long since by the announcement of the discovery of a new bacterial organism as the cause of cancer.   For the past fifteen years the discovery of some bacterial organism associated with cancer has been an annual event. During that same period hardly a month has passed by but what the editor of *The Journal of the American Medical Association* has had submitted to him manuscripts advancing new theories as to the cause of this malignant condition, and not the least among these theories have been those associated with dietary fallacies. In England the exploiters of this peculiar idea have been such men as the surgeon, Arbuthnot Lane, and the publicist, J. E. Barker. Indeed, even Sir Clifford Allbut before his death was drawn into the controversy in the support of whole wheat bread as contrasted with that made from white flour. It was Sir Clifford Allbut's view that the whole wheat flour was richer, that it had a more agreeable flavor than the white loaf, which he said was insipid, and that the vitamins are illusive and must be sought in the whole grain. Once this view was advanced, others came to its support and medical health officers and general practitioners did not hesitate to advance their opinions. Arbuthnot Lane committed himself some years ago to the view that most of the ills of mankind are caused by intestinal stasis or constipation. He urged the use of whole wheat bread to relieve constipation and he short-circuited the intestines and removed their kinks as a quick surgical road to the relief sought. It was a witty American surgeon who commented: "It's a long lane that has no kink."

As might have been expected, it was not long before the British hyperenthusiasm infected the United States. Among the first to seize upon this conception for journalistic exploitation was the organ of that most erudite of automobile manufacturers, Mr. Henry Ford. The man, who found difficulty in distinguishing between Benedict Arnold and Arnold Bennett, did not hesitate, through the periodical that he sponsors, to support the view that the eating of white flour bread is responsible for cancer. There was about as much actual knowledge behind the latter opinion as behind the former. There is not an iota of scientific evidence that the eating of white bread, or any other kind of bread, will cause cancer, and not the slightest reason to believe that the use of whole wheat bread will in any way prevent it.

Before making a definite statement as to the actual value of white flour bread as contrasted with whole wheat, it should be emphasized again that neither white flour bread nor whole wheat bread constitutes a single article in diet for any intelligent person. As pointed out by McCollum, there are many reasons why the American can eat white flour bread satisfactorily. "White flour," he says, "keeps much better than whole wheat flour and so can be handled with less commercial hazard. The American public likes white flour bread, and I do not see any reason," he continues, "why this taste should be disturbed. The important thing is to insist upon the consumption of a sufficient amount of what I have termed the protective foods—milk and vegetables of the leafy type—to insure that calcium deficiency and the vitamin deficiency of white bread will be made good." If baking technologic research is able to incorporate larger amounts of milk solids in the loaf of bread or otherwise to insure a sufficient amount of calcium and the important vitamins, even this charge cannot rest against white flour bread.

The supporters of whole wheat as against white flour for dietary purposes argue that the human bowel requires a certain amount of roughage in order to exercise its functions satisfactorily. This point must not be considered without reference to the varying conditions that may exist in different individuals. Dr. W. C. Alvarez of the Hooper Foundation for Medical Research has vigorously attacked the unguarded and unqualified recommendation of coarse food substances. "Some men and women can be greatly helped by bran," he says, "and their constipation can be cured if they happen to have the digestion of an ostrich; but if they happen to have congenitally defective or handicapped digestive tracts; if they have ulcers or narrow places, they cannot handle the mass of indigestible material and they promptly get into trouble." Many other dietary substances such as celery, lettuce, spinach and raisins provide roughage. Why ask bread to be like Messalina, all things to all men? It is for the individual physician, knowing the condition of the intestinal tract of the person with whom he is especially concerned to determine whether or not that person ought to use breads or other foods that depart from the standard product or from the normal diet. For those who do not have such special recommendation, the standard white bread loaf, that forms the large portion of bread baked in the United States to-day, is the product to be recommended as most satisfactory.

We are a people singularly cursed with faddists. We have educational cults, healing cults, religious cults and heaven alone knows how many peculiar promotional systems. We have dietary faddists who believe that the eating of more white bread, more wheat, more fruit or more raisins is necessary to healthful living. The time has arrived for calling a halt to the growing procession of slogans that tend to promote panaceas for health and well-being. We are admonished at every turn to eat more bread, to drink more milk, to buy more raisins, to consume more apples, to confine ourselves to whole wheat, to try some bran, or to add one or another of a dozen different items to our daily regimen. Many persons have a limited tolerance for a food like raisins and the victim of chronic inflammation of the intestines may hesitate to secure his iron through a "mixture of sugar and skins" as one caustic commentor characterized this confection.

The starchy foods, wheat, corn, rice and potatoes, are universal sources of food for the body. Bread, the very staff of life, gives that feeling of satisfaction following eating that is an important factor in a suitable diet. One should not urge the sedentary, the desk-ridden or any other muscularly inactive person to eat more meat or more wheat or to increase his bread supply.   Americans to-day tend more and more to suffer with obesity or overweight. It is the opinion of those best informed that over-weight is one of the most important factors in shortening the span of human life.   Physiologists have established the fact that a meal composed largely of cereals is passed through the stomach within one and a half hours, whereas the inclusion of meat will prolong the time two or three hours. In recommending a diet of cereals and starchy foods as compared with meats, fats and cheese, these things must be taken into account by the physician.

Conclusion

The scientific physician welcomes the establish-ment of a standard loaf of bread made according to the best scientific evidence as to what is de-manded in bread by the taste of the public, by our knowledge of nutrition and of the mysterious vita mins.   Such a product can be included in diets both for the sick and for the well with a clear under-standing of the effect that it may have on digestion and growth.   The physician opposes the promotion of any single article of diet according to "the all or nothing policy" as the one substance important to health or the control of disease.   In efforts at education of the public, which the modern physi-cian believes is the most important factor in lengthening the span of life, faddist notions must be attacked with all the vigor and influence that the scientific pen can command either by purchase of advertising space or by the contribution of articles published for the public good. The time is near at hand when the compliment given by Don Quixote to a knight of his acquaintance may be used without fear of attack from any meticulous critic. The Don remarked to his squire, Sancho Panza: "He is as good as good bread."

CHAPTER VII

THE END OF ECLECTICISM

I

IN books on medical history the term Eclecticism has two meanings. The first goes back to the Greeks. Following the collection of the Hippocratic texts before the Christian era, certain Greek physicians and scientists formed a group of Eclectics who proposed to dispense with preconceived notions and to develop a school of scientific medicine. But they passed, and from the period of Galen (200 A.D.) until that of Paracelsus (1493-1541 A.D.) medicine rested in oblivion while men gave more thought to their souls than to their bodies, to argument than to observation, to theory than to scientific fact.

Then came the second Eclecticism. The biting sarcasm of Paracelsus disturbed the calm belief in Galenic medicine, and the discoveries of Vesalius in anatomy, of Harvey as to the circulation of blood, of Jenner concerning vaccination, and particularly of Leeuwenhoek, maker of microscopes, restored accurate observation to its proper leading position in the science of medicine. But the new methods brought new enthusiasts, and a host of new systems threatened to impede all actual progress. Mesmerism, Brunonianism, phrenology, homeopathy, Rade-

macherism, Baunscheidtism, hydropathy, odic force
and animal magnetism contended for favor and
scentific inquiry was neglected. The appeal of
the bizarre is strong even to enlightened men; to
a public educated to a belief in the black art,
magic, alchemy and the miracles of the saints, the
unusual necessarily had an absolute fascination.
Medicine in this way became inordinately complex
and chaotic.

Into this maze came Christian Wilhelm Hufeland, whose whole career was a protest against the
confusion. To him systems of medicine were anathema. He wanted the facts. With the founding
of his *Journal of Practical Medicine* in 1795 there
began a battle for the scientific study of disease
that is still going on. Of him it may be said that
he was truly eclectic. And after Hufeland came
Canstatt, Wunderlich, Skoda, Rokitansky and all
those other robust German scientists who laid the
foundations of modern medicine.

But what of American Eclecticism? What relation did it have to Hufeland and his work? And
what has become of it? Medical historians at home
apparently take but little pride in it, and foreign
historians seem to be unaware of its existence.
Even the erudite Fielding H. Garrison, whose "History of Medicine" is the last word in English on the
subject, astutely ignores this Eclecticism. In what
is perhaps his only reference to it he waxes, for so
calm a man, a little acrid. "In America, under

existing legislation," he affirms, "every species of medical sect—osteopathy, chiropraxis, Christian Science, eclecticism, botanic medicine, etc.—has been permitted to flourish."

In the land of the free Eclecticism is thus something different. It is a system of medicine which treats disease by the application of single remedies to known disturbances, without reference to any scientific classification, but giving special attention to the development of plant remedies. It is the apotheosis of the old grandmother and witch-doctor systems of treatment. It arose out of the attempts of a widow to conserve her husband's income and out of the medical practice of an old-woman herb doctor. It profited and prospered, no doubt, by that same reaction against the drastic *materia medica* of the period around the year 1800 that gave us homeopathy.

Those were days of heavy drugging. Dr. Benjamin Rush, one of the signers of the Declaration of Independence, was equally well known, in medical circles at least, as the designer of a purgative combination of jalap and calomel so potent as to merit the title of Rush's Thunderbolt. Homeopathy owed its initial success to the fact that it prescribed small doses of remedies in vast quantities of water, and so did not interfere with the natural tendency of the body to recover. On this tendency—the *vis medicatrix naturæ*—all of the cults of history have floated their frail vessels. Eclecticism did so like the rest. It discarded most of the mineral remedies of the time and emphasized the use of the milder drugs derived from plants. It urged the use of single remedies and at most of simple combinations. Since most of the remedies it promoted have since been shown to be quite inert or utterly inadequate in the large majority of cases, the vogue of the cult must have rested on the same desire to escape over-drugging that promoted homeopathy. And it had a vogue! At the height of that vogue it graduated several hundred physicians every year from ten medical colleges. But gradually, as scientific medicine progressed, its ranks dwindled, and it fell into the hands of exploiters and promoters. To-day it totters feebly in one recognized school and in several diploma mills, it finds itself involved in noisome licensure scandals, and it is likely to succumb shortly to what physicians in their consultations call an *exitus lethalis*.

2

Dr. George Andrew Viesselius, born in Holland (or Germany), emigrated to this country in 1749, settled in New Jersey, married an American girl and established a comfortable practice. When he died in 1767 there remained on his estate, in addition to his widow, a bound or hired boy named Jacob Tidd. Jacob used to help the doctor out by making up washes, salves, plasters and similar

external applications according to formulæ that
Viesselius had brought from abroad. The community boasted few practitioners and when Viesselius died the widow, as is not unusual with widows,
decided to keep the practice going with the assistance of Jacob Tidd. Jacob came into possession,
through this association, of the professional papers
of Doctor Viesselius. In 1796-1800 he was in
Western Pennsylvania for a time. It is not re-
corded whether he served as an army doctor or as
a private soldier during the Whisky Insurrection,
although he did serve, but it is noted that he secured
herb remedies from the Indians directly and also
from a relative who had been a captive among them.

Returning from the war, Tidd set up as a doctor
at Ringoes, New Jersey, and soon acquired a lucra-
tive practice. For forty years he practiced at Am-
well, in Hunterdon County, New Jersey, apparently
limiting himself largely to the external remedies
that were a heritage from the old Dutch doctor.
Many persons came to him to learn his methods and
among them was one Wooster Beach. Beach was
born in Trumbull, Connecticut, in 1794. He educated himself and his biographers relate that he
pursued eagerly all the adverse criticisms on the
medicine of the time that came his way. One day
he heard about Jacob Tidd, and went to him in
search of instruction. "Suspicious lest his means
of livelihood would be wrested from him," says the
biographer, "he [Tidd] flatly refused to receive

Beach, as he had many others who had applied for the same privilege." Here is one of the marks of the charlatan in medicine. The true medical scientist has no secrets that he guards from other physicians; his knowledge is broadcast through the medical periodicals so that physicians everywhere may use it in alleviating the ills of mankind.

Let us see the type of energy that inspired Beach. In a letter he said: "I was obliged to return home disappointed. But the same anxiety continued, and I felt, respecting my one desire, something as the Apostle Paul is represented to have felt respecting religion, when he said, 'A dispensation of the gospel is committed unto me, and woe be unto me if I preach not the gospel.'" Of such stuff are the founders of cults made; one always finds them prating in terms of theological derivation, and usually affirming their ability to commune personally with the Deity. Again and again Beach attempted to study with Jacob Tidd. Finally, he came at a time when Tidd was without an assistant. Beach took the place and remained until Tidd died at seventy-four years of age; then he succeeded to the practice. Beach was the formulator of Eclecticism—first under the name of the Reformed Practice of Medicine.

Eventually he went to New York, to treat several cases to which he was called in consultation. He settled there and is said to have become belatedly a student at a medical college, graduating in

due form and becoming a member of the New York
County Medical Society. In 1825 he started teach-
ing and writing, attacking the use of blood-letting
and strong remedies and urging his students to treat
disease with nature's remedies—herbs and roots.
In 1827 he opened an infirmary in Eldridge Street,
New York, and in 1837 he started the New York
Medical Academy, which eventually became the
Reformed Medical College of New York, the
parent school of the Eclectic system.

In the meantime, the system of practice known
as Thomsonism, later incorporated into Eclecticism,
had been developing independently. Samuel Thomson was born in New Hampshire in 1769. When
he was four years old he discovered that lobelia,
or Indian tobacco (*Lobelia inflata*), an indigenous
herb, if chewed, induced vomiting. He amused himself by getting his boy friends to chew it. An old
woman herbalist in the vicinity told him more about
roots and grasses. He tried to study medicine under
a root doctor near by, but was refused owing to his
deficient education. Then he married, went to
farming and began a family. One of his children
fell ill of scarlet fever and when the attending physician gave up the case Thomson tried steam in-
halations and lobelia with success. Then he became
a traveling herb doctor and had his remedies pat-
ented in Washington. It will be remembered,
perhaps, that the rise of osteopathy hinged on the
death of one of the daughters of Andrew Still.

Eventually Thomson tried to settle down in Massachusetts, but he was bitterly attacked by the local medical profession as a quack. Once he was acquitted of murdering some one with too much lobelia; after the trial he found that he had earned sufficient popularity to encourage him to open an office in Boston. The Thomson system of treating disease with herbs, mostly lobelia, was taken up to some extent by others and flourished for twenty years. Thomson died in 1843 "heroically partaking of his own remedies until the very end." His "New Guide to Health," written in 1822, passed through many editions, and at last became "Thomson's Materia Medica or Botanic Family Physician." Although opposed by Wooster Beach, who was little inclined to welcome competition, Thomsonism soon became incorporated into the Eclectic system.

On May 3, 1830, the Reformed Medical Society of New York, founded to support the ideas and the school of Beach, adopted a resolution to found an additional school of Eclectic medicine in some town on the Ohio River. It was hoped that in the newly opened country better opportunity would exist for the new school to lead an untrammeled existence. The school was established at Worthington, Ohio, in 1833, as the Worthington Medical College, but it did not thrive. It suspended its sessions in 1839. In 1843 it removed to Cincinnati, which is still the fountain-head of Eclecticism in this country. In 1845 it became the Eclectic Medical Institute. By

1848 it was again in difficulties and a convention was called in Cincinnati to organize a national society of Eclectic practitioners. Wooster Beach's name headed the list of organizers, and in 1855 the grand old man of Eclecticism became the president of this society.

In the meantime disciples of Eclecticism had been spreading the gospel hither and thither in our fair land. Colleges rose and fell like the flowers that bloom in the spring. The New York Reformed Medical College, born in 1826, was extinct about 1839. The College of Medicine, Botanic, organized in New York City in 1836, died in 1846. The Eclectic Medical Institute of New York, created in 1847 as the Medical School of Fredonia, moved to Rochester in 1848, merged with the Randolph Eclectic Medical Institute and moved to Syracuse in 1849 and became the Central Medical College of New York. In 1850 it moved back to Rochester and in 1852 it had its *exitus lethalis*. The Eclectic Medical College of New York City, organized in 1866, graduated its first class in 1867 and then sent forth one every year until 1913, when it succumbed. In the early days running a medical college was usually a profitable procedure, and was thus considered an important accessory to medical practice.

So the colleges of Eclectic medicine came and went. The facts for New York were duplicated on a smaller scale in other States, but a multiplication of examples is needless. In 1860 there were four

Eclectic medical colleges, and they graduated some two hundred dispensers of plant remedies. In 1870 there were five schools, in 1880 eight and in 1890 and in 1900 nine. Shortly after this time the Council on Medical Education of the American Medical Association began its investigative and publicity activities. At once the number of Eclectic schools and the number of their graduates began to decline. By 1915 there were but four Eclectic schools, and since 1920 there has remained but one, the school in Cincinnati supported by the National Eclectic Medical Association. True, the Kansas City College of Medicine and Surgery has claimed to be Eclectic, but the National Eclectic Association disowns it and it finds itself of late involved in a diploma-mill scandal. In 1925 the Cincinnati school gave but thirty-eight graduates to the world. Its complete enrollment was one hundred and forty-eight students. Its average attendance during the last five years has been about one hundred.

3

During the craze for the development of botanical drugs our pharmacopeia became almost a replica of the herbals of seventeenth and eighteenth century Europe. The woods and the fields were combed for all varieties of roots and vines and grasses, and they were transformed into infusions, decoctions, syrups, tinctures, extracts and tablets. The mind of the poor medical student was bewildered by .his attempts to learn the botanical names, the nature, and the alleged uses of these hundreds of drugs. Into this confusion the Council on Pharmacy and Chemistry swept like a tempest, supported by blasts from the university laboratories which were carefully investigating, on animals and on man, the real virtues of the remedies in use. Far-seeing practitioners like William Osler were condemning the superfluity of preparations, and urging the use only of such as were actually capable of producing definite effects in definite dosages. That the plant remedies survived at all was due not so much to the efforts of the Eclectic colleges as to the manufacturers of Eclectic remedies and, above all, to the promoters of patent medicines, which were composed largely of complex mixtures of such substances—veritable vegetable soups.

A report of the Council on Pharmacy and Chemistry on one of these Eclectic remedies is typical of what has been done to hundreds of them. *Echinacea angustefolia* was first introduced as the main ingredient of a remedy known as Meyer's Blood Purifier. This preparation, according to the label, was powerful as an alterative and antiseptic in all "tumorous and syphilitic indications, old chronic wounds such as fever sores, old ulcers, carbuncles, piles, eczema, wet or dry, also erysipelas and gangrene." It was also "a specific for fever," "ad-

verted typhoid in two or three days," and cured
malaria, malignant, remittent and mountain fever,
diphtheria, bites "from the bee to the rattlesnake,"
and mad dog bites. Obviously a medical gem! The
drug was promptly adopted by the medicos of
the Eclectic school, and shortly afterward different
proprietary concerns introduced it to the public
under the names of echtisia, ecthol and echitone.
Echtisia contained, in addition to the echinacea,
some wild indigo, arbor vitæ and poke root; and
echitone contained also pansy and blue flag. The
company promoting the former asserted that wild
indigo was a "destroyer of devitalizing elements
in the blood" and a "vitalizer of the blood as well,"
that arbor vitæ was "a perfect antiseptic and a gen-
erator of vital force in disorganized tissues" and
that a long list of diseases, including diphtheria,
syphilitic sciatica and gonorrheal rheumatism, were
"all more or less amenable to full doses" of poke
root.

All of this was, of course, the veriest bosh. For
the conditions mentioned scientific medicine has provided methods of treatment and remedies that attack the cause. For scarlet fever it has an anti-
toxin and it disregards the *rhus toxicodendron* of
the Eclectic pharmacopeia; for angina pectoris it
seeks sedation and attempts by intricate surgical
methods to cut off the sensations of pain, discarding
the "specific medicine lobelia" of the Eclectics as an
unreliable and poisonous drug. The recommenda-

tion of bryonia for pain over the eye regardless of the cause, of spigelia for headache over the top of the head increasing in the morning and decreasing in the afternoon, of cactus and white hellebore and gelsemium for oppressive pain on the top of the head caused by uterine displacement—all of these recommendations, taken from the guide-books of Eclectic medicine, scientific medicine greets to-day with laughter.

"Slowly, but surely, botanical drugs, upon which many packaged medicines rely for their therapeutic benefits and for the therapeutic claim made for them, are being dropped from the United States Pharmacopœia," says an editorial in the October, 1925, number of *Standard Remedies,* the official organ of the package medicine industry. "Seventeen such drugs were dropped from the 1920 revision of the Pharmacopœia just issued. In 1910 twenty-two were dropped. In 1900 eleven were dropped. The few remaining may be dropped in the next or some future revision." And in an article in the same issue Mr. H. C. Fuller says: "Publications of the Eclectic School still support many of the therapeutic claims that have been advanced for a large number of botanical drugs that appear in the above list. However, even here we find a tendency to conservatism and at times a repudiation of earlier opinions."

Mr. Fuller, a friend of the package medicine industry, views this situation with alarm. "It is coming to pass," he says, "that the deletion of botanical drugs from official standards and the omission of references to their therapeutic value in modern text-books, as well as definite statements discrediting the former ideas of their efficacy, will eventually bring about the situation that preparations containing these drugs will have no standing or authoritative support, and will be thrown back almost solely on testimonials, which experience has demonstrated are often of doubtful value. The preparations chiefly affected at present are the so-called Blood Remedies or Alteratives, Rheumatism Remedies, Kidney Remedies, Female Remedies and Nerve Remedies." Here is a statement from an expert as to the present low state of botanical remedies! Mr. Fuller suggests to the manufacturers that the proper procedure would be the employment of research with a view to reëstablishing in good scientific usage the remedies which constitute the basis of their nostrums. But do not think Mr. Fuller is naïve; the available information indicates that he is prepared to promote such researches at a reasonable figure.

Thus all the signs and portents indicate that the great deluge of modern scientific chemotherapy is about to wash away the plant and vegetable débris. With that washing will go the last vestiges of Thomsonism and the Eclectic practice of Wooster Beach.

4

As I have said, the number of medical schools in the United States began to increase rapidly after the Civil War. The creation of many of these schools was due to the self-interest of the men constituting their faculties. Money was to be made by teaching students, and prestige was to be acquired by a self-conferred title of professor. The standards of medical education in this country thus became an offense in the sight of the leaders of American medicine. With the advent of each new medical cult and of each new group of medical colleges devoted to it, the State legislatures were besought to create separate boards of examiners for the licensing of graduates.

Obviously, the medical practice laws in all the States are intended to safeguard the public against incompetent and untrained physicians. Where States have but a single board administering the act it accomplishes that purpose. Unfortunately, when new boards are created for various new types of practitioners, the medical practice acts are promptly nullified. If there is such a thing as scientific medicine, and if there are diseases such as smallpox, tuberculosis, typhoid fever and measles which produce definite changes in the human body, every one who wants to treat human disease ought to be able to recognize the changes they bring about, to diag-

nose them when present and to know how to prescribe preventive measures to keep them from
spreading throughout the community.   Certainly
every one who wants to practice the healing art by
any method of treatment should be willing to come
before an examining body and give evidence of his
knowledge of these fundamental things.   Nevertheless, the legislators in the various States have
created ninety-six separate and independent boards
to control medical licensure in America.   In some
States there are actually five or six different boards
created by as many independent medical practice
acts, and vesting as many different standards of
educational qualification.

Out of this confused mass of laws came a great
licensure scandal in 1923, and in that scandal Eclectic medical boards played the most prominent part.
In 1918, five years before, the *Journal of the
American Medical Association* had protested against
the manner in which graduates of low-grade medical
colleges in Missouri were being licensed by the
Eclectic boards in Arkansas and Connecticut.   For
the next five years, it published annually a protest,
and indeed insinuated definitely that neither the
Arkansas State Board of Eclectic Examiners nor
the Kansas City, Missouri, College of Medicine and
Surgery could exist unless they were in cahoots.
Connecticut, too, was warned again and again that
it was harboring a menace in its Eclectic board.
But in 1920 the Kansas City College and the

Arkansas Eclectic Board entente was still doing business, the former graduating thirty-three men and the latter licensing all but one of them, and in 1921 the Missouri legislature removed the word "reputable," as it related to medical colleges, from its medical practice act and substituted the words, "legally chartered."

In 1922 there developed a new entente: the Connecticut board licensed seventy-one physicians, sixty-one of whom graduated from low-grade medical colleges and three from institutions in California which apparently had never been recognized as professional schools of any type. Of the seventy-one medicos licensed in Connecticut, only twenty-five had actually graduated from Eclectic medical colleges, but forty-six more, who logically should have applied to the so-called regular medical board, since they had graduated from what were presumably regular medical colleges, although of extremely low standing, apparently had arranged with the Eclectic board in Connecticut to provide them with licenses. The situation, uncovered first by the St. Louis *Star,* showed clearly that graduates of the St. Louis College of Physicians and Surgeons were being shipped to Connecticut so that the Connecticut Eclectic board might give them legal entrance into the practice of medicine. The reciprocity laws between the various States then permitted them to ooze gradually out of Connecticut and into other communities.

Following the investigation of 1923, the licenses of one hundred and sixty-seven physicians who had been certified by the Connecticut Eclectic board were revoked, but seventy-three of these physicians were allowed to continue to practice until their cases are heard by the superior courts. Any one conversant with legal procedure may figure out how long it will be until the Supreme Court acts on these cases and confirms the revocations of licenses. But Eclecticism meanwhile is gasping out its last breaths. It was ill for a long time; now a lethal draught of scandal has finished it.

Thus the growth of cults within the science of medicine provided opportunity for evading the requirement of certain fundamental knowledge in those who proposed to deal with the ailments of humanity. In that evasion the separate State boards dealing with Eclecticism seem to have played a most prominent part. The only hope for the protection of the public against such dubious cultists lies in having but one board of medical examiners in each State, and in establishing one minimum standard of qualifications to which every one must measure who is to have the legal right to practice healing. The exemptions of cults because they limit their methods of treatment to manipulation, to mental suggestion, to plant remedies, to highly diluted remedies, or to any other quackery is merely throwing open the doors to unqualified, incompetent, mendacious and unprincipled pretenders.

CHAPTER VIII

PHYSICAL AND ELECTRIC THERAPY

THE editor's occupation affords him opportunity
to display either broad and comprehensive ignorance or erudite knowledge of many topics before
audiences composed of specialists in various fields.
Following his glittering generalizations he is likely
to become the recipient of anathema and vitupera-
tion for his disagreements with long-held opinions.
Obviously, the knowledge of physical therapy which
forms the basis of the considerations here presented
is not derived from personal observation of the
devices used in physical therapy, from an intimate
study of their effects on animals or on patients, or
even from their trial on a physical constitution
inured to punishment by the trials of numerous
toothpastes, breakfast foods, condensed, dried and
powdered milks, or other samples conferred on
editors by earnest manufacturers and a progressive
advertising department. Such statements as are
here made public result from the reading of in-
numerable manuscripts submitted by aspirants for
fame in the field of physical therapy; from the re-
viewing of a considerable number of major opuses
that have emanated from the pens of physical
therapeutic scribes—some obviously, some possibly,

some ostensibly, and some not likely in the employ of concerns producing apparatus; from conferences with many specialists in this growing field, and, finally, from an attempt to apply to the assembled information what is known as editorial judgment— a thing sometimes called by cynics the result of a disordered digestion.

No doubt the first agents of treatment used by man were those which could be had through simple adaptations of things natural. The application of heat and cold, rubbing and massage, and the use of water and of sunlight are as old as man himself. In the aphorisms of Hippocrates one reads of the uses of such methods; even at that time sound observers seem to have realized that these agents may act for good or for evil.

"Heat is suppurative," says one aphorism, "but not in all kinds of sores; but when it is, it furnishes the greatest test of their being free from danger. It softens the skin, makes it thin, removes pain, soothes rigor, convulsions and tetanus." But again, "Heat produces the following bad effects on those who use it frequently: enervation of the fleshy parts, impotence of the nerves, torpor of the understanding, hemorrhages, .deliquia, and along with these, death." And in commenting on the latter aphorism, Galen and, still later, Celsus, said: "By 'heat' is meant 'hot water' or a 'hot fomentation.'"

Massage, too, was practiced in the earliest times: Anthropologists and ethnologists have described the practice as it exists among savage peoples to-day, and accounts are found in primitive medical texts. It is repeatedly referred to in the folk-lore of all nations, particularly in the tales of the Arabian Nights. Such massage included not only simple rubbing, but also pinching and kneading, later classified by French and Swedish investigators with technical terms.

The ancient Egyptians, the Greeks and the Romans were firm believers in the health-giving powers of the sun's rays. Indeed, Herodotus asserted that light must be regarded by the physician who knows his business as a means of repelling illness and as a subsequent aid to recovery. There were sun rooms in the homes of all the well-to-do Romans, not glassed-in sun-parlors facing north, as in our apartments to-day, but large central spaces, open to the sky and to the sun itself.

Humphris tells us that the first use of electricity in healing took place in the time of Tiberius, some twenty years after the death of Christ, when a physician named Scribonius Largus made use of the Raja torpedo-fish for rheumatism and for headaches. The electric ray-fish and the electric eel of Brazil are said to be able to convey a considerable shock. Scribonius Largus was, however, known chiefly for the scope of his writings, as his name no doubt indicates. His recommendation was based, apparently, wholly on empiricism. Much the same sort of reasoning assigned unusual virtues to mixtures of drugs of foul smell or of nauseous taste. The results commonly are the proof of the power of suggestion.

Of the birth of the roentgen ray and of the finer electric apparatus of our modern times, accurate descriptions are easily available. From the primitive observations of the past have arisen these remarkably complicated devices that have made necessary increased knowledge by the physician of physics and of chemistry, of physiology and of biology, and that call for a finer discrimination in their choice and in their application to disease than it has been necessary to accord to many of the drugs used in medicine.

SCIENCE VERSUS EMPIRICISM

The proper evaluation of evidence regarding the use of new methods in the treatment of disease is difficult. The patient is anxious to be well, the physician wants to see him cured or at least benefited as promptly as possible, and his friends and relatives constantly endeavor to encourage him, regardless of their actual belief as to the state of his illness. The result of this continuous positive suggestion is to lend to any method of treatment that may be employed a credence that is perhaps not its actual due. Few physicians—and, indeed, few scientists—can resist the hyperenthusiasm that is likely to follow a first successful result. The paths of the history of therapy are bestrewn with the wrecks of new cures that sailed forth as the last word in therapeutic achievement. Mental, manipulative, natural, mystical, spiritual and other cures have been brought forth by apostles of healing and vaunted as the secret for the solution of all the problems of healing that have confronted the physician since the earliest times. But when the apostle died, or when the primal faith that animated his followers disappeared, the cure went the way of the apostle.

Now physical therapy has been more subject to misunderstanding of its efficacy in varied conditions than has any other form used by the scientific physician. The potency of the placebo depends only on the mental suggestion and on the personality of the man who administers it. His contact with the patient is not direct. The contact of the chiropractor, the osteopath and the religious healer consists usually of the direct laying on of hands. Few physicians of experience fail to realize the importance of such immediate relationship to the patient. If more physicians took the trouble to make thorough examinations of their patients, never failing to examine the chest after the clothing had been completely removed from the upper part of the body and using auscultation, percussion and palpation, which are fundamental to physical diagnosis, there would be fewer failures and many more persons satisfied with the care of their physicians.

Without doubt, powerful suggestion is conveyed by the use of any intricate or striking mechanical method. The use of electricity, including the direct application of the current, the galvanic apparatus, pocket batteries and all the assorted forms of waves supplied through more intricate mechanisms, as well as the use of electricity to produce heat and light, is a striking therapeutic procedure. The late—but not too late—Albert Abrams well knew the value of intricate apparatus for impressing the patient and, even more, for impressing the uncritical physician. His first venture, spondylotherapy, carried with it a physically intensified suggestion; and those later Goldbergian evolvements, the oscilloclast and the biodynamometer, were impressive in their complexity even to some competent physicians.

Regardless of the fact that the underlying basis for many physical methods never has been thoroughly established and, indeed, is not even yet perfectly understood, the official organ of the American Electrotherapeutic Association only recently said: "The various irregular cults have also worked out in some instances methods that have sometimes succeeded where the rank and file of the medical profession have failed." The editorial referred to cites particularly the treatment of sacro-iliac strain, recommending, first, adjustment and, secondly, the application of electricity. On what basis does the editorial presume to say that displaced vertebræ once adjusted remain adjusted, unless held in place

over long periods of time by methods of fixation?
Who has proved that ligaments that are relaxed will
resume their functions when the supposed luxations
are properly replaced? Who has made the scientific studies, using the roentgen ray and all the other
methods known to modern science, by which even
an iota of truth can be attached to the claims of
chiropractic and, indeed, to most of those of osteopathy? Granting that there is a modicum of truth
in the claims of the latter cult, what scientific organization will be willing to admit that half-educated
and incompetent men with no thorough understanding of the human body and its mechanisms should be
privileged to apply any single form of therapy or
diagnosis?

The Dangers of Systems and Specialties

If medicine is to be partitioned off into a series
of specialties and cults practiced by men who have
learned only one organ of the body or only one
system of diagnosing and of treating disease, medicine as a science is bound to fail. No part of the
human body can be detached and treated as separate
from the organism as a whole. This danger threatens all the forms of physical therapy. It was no
doubt enthusiasm for a single method that caused an
editorial writer in the official organ of electrotherapy to say that "physical therapy will ultimately
be recognized as of greater value than all other

therapeutic methods." This concentration on an "all or nothing" policy in the treatment of disease must inevitably lead to preposterous and exaggerated claims, and ultimately to the detriment of scientific practice. Physicians have watched the inroads made on the practice of medicine as a single science. They have noted the attempts of optometrists to parcel off the eye as their particular field; of cosmeticians to assume the right to treat disorders of the skin and to request legislatures to grant them power to remove moles, warts, tumors and other excrescences; of chiropodists to assign to themselves the complete care of the feet; of chiropractors and osteopaths to make the field of manual manipulation their exclusive purview; and of some of the specialists within the ranks of medicine itself to assign all important functions to the teeth, to the lungs or to other organs of the body. The time has come to call a halt on geographic warfare within the human body, and to look on it as a "united states" that will be at least as firmly consolidated as the forty-eight individual constituents of our government.

If electrotherapy could point to a past that was free from the faults that have marred the progress of drug therapy since the earliest times, it would need no caution as to the future. But what has become of the hundreds of galvanic apparatus that struck amazement to the hearts of trembling children led into physicians' offices some twenty-five years ago? Where are the little electric batteries that formerly occupied the showcases in the drug stores? Indeed, what has become of the claims for high voltage roentgen ray in the removal of deep-seated malignancy? What a brief period it required for these claims, vaunted as the last word in the control of cancer, to resolve themselves into a method used only in apparently hopeless cases! The judgment may be premature, but it is based on scientific studies made in well-recognized institutions for the study of human diseases.

PHYSICAL THERAPY PROMOTION

There was a time when the medical scientist, having completed his education in the field to which he wished to devote himself, opened his office, began teaching in a medical school with which he had affiliated himself, undertook the care of patients in legitimate hospitals, and left it to the recognition of the public to advance him to the limit of his merits. To-day, modern high-powered business methods applied to the practice of medicine have pointed the way to the cults and to the hyperenthusiastic practitioner for promotion of his particular plans. All the forces of publicity are directed toward urging on the public the peculiar advantages that are claimed to accrue to single methods. The high priest of the peculiar system does not hesitate to instruct his followers in promotion of the system by all the arts and crafts—mostly the crafts—of salesmanship. There are physical therapists who believe that "high frequency" means the treatment of eighty patients a day. Again, organizations are established, not for study and investigation or for the promotion of knowledge in relation to the growth of any department of medical science, but primarily for the securing of public acclaim through the organization, rather than through the individual. The multiplicity of medical organizations is evidence of the fact that in some instances they are not established with investigation and study as their main objects. Consider in this connection the society called the Association for Medico-Physical Research. In its meeting, one program is devoted entirely to the claims of the now discredited Abrams method; another, to the exploitation of methods for the treatment of cancer, not one of which is established on any sort of a sound foundation; and still others to the promotion of systems of practice that should meet with nothing but the scorn of all who consider themselves honest and ethical practitioners of medicine. One finds here names of men known as faddists, who have discarded scientific rationality. One, without regard to the established facts of science, insists that a rice diet will prevent and cure cancer. Another promotes the treatment of cancer with a serum, regardless of the fact that carefully made investigations have revealed the failure of his method. There is G. E. Harter of the Defensive Diet League of America, who has collected a lot of miscellaneous aphorisms and peculiar concepts concerning food into a system and who has inveigled dentists of this country to his support with the idea that it is the duty of the dentists to establish the food habits of the nation. Among this miscellaneous crew of peculiar faddists appear the names of some physicians whose places on the program apparently represent an attempt to camouflage, with a sort of medical aristocracy, the fallacies that occupy the major portion of the program.

Basis of Physical Therapy

The results of physical therapy seem to depend on many factors. Without doubt, rays of light have many and varying effects on the human body. Attempts have been made to separate them into effects of the light itself on the tissues and into chemical effects. Electricity has the power of acting through the heat that may be produced and, perhaps, through some effects produced by the current itself not yet determined; indeed, the mechanism is no better determined than is that of immunity in general. Electric stimulation no doubt has the power to act on nerves and on muscles, producing visible motive effects; and with such effects come mechanical changes. Is it not time that intensive study be applied in an analytic manner to determine to just what extent the benefits observed from the various electrotherapeutic measures are due to physical changes in the tissues, to mechanical changes in the tissues, to the power of suggestion, and, perhaps, to other factors of which we know nothing? Until some adequate basis on which the methods may rest is determined, no one can call such methods truly scientific. We have in physical therapy various methods of producing heat in the human body. There is the heat produced by friction; the heat produced by the external application of light, of hot water or of other heat-producing methods; and the heat produced within the body by diathermy, by the direct injection of heating material, or by the use of methods that will draw unusual quantities of blood to a certain point. In the evaluation of any form of physical therapy, who shall say to what extent the thermic factor alone is responsible and how far the other factors that have been mentioned have a part to play?

The numerous devices for effecting the production of heat, external or internal, for the body unquestionably vary in their potency and in their mechanism. How is the individual physician who knows little or nothing of the physical basis of electricity and, in fact, who knows little or nothing of any physics at all, except in the use of the term as it applies to castor oil and cascara, to have any actual knowledge of these so-called modalities?

Drug products are compounds of chemical substances and may easily be separated into their individual ingredients. Scientific pharmacy has already made sufficient progress to warrant the statement that these ingredients will or will not do what is claimed for them. But when one is confronted with a large box beautifully trimmed with nickel plate and glass, the interior of which is a mass of wiring, spools, coils, gages, screws, nuts and what not, and is told that, properly applied, this apparatus will cure pneumonia, neuritis, lumbago, eczema, dysmenorrhea, falling of the uterus and falling of the palate, who is to tell one whether or not the machine will actually do all that is claimed for it? When the text-books in the field of physical therapy tell the physician that the spine of the patient with locomotor ataxia may be restored to its pristine glory by running a few shocks up and down from the cervical region to the coccyx, is he to discard the prognosis that he has made in the past and to tell the friends and relatives of the victim of the wiles of Venus that his lapse from virtue is to have no further evil effects? What is the physician to do when he learns that most of the text-books in this field are the products of men who are employed by concerns selling apparatus; when he is constantly besieged with lecture courses paid for by those who have something to sell; when his office is inundated with literature telling him that his financial future depends on the purchase of a vast amount of such machinery? Clearly, a housecleaning is badly needed in this particular field.

The advance of electrotherapeutics under the guidance of its pioneers was an enthusiastic but bitter warfare against a stubborn and conservative medical profession. The introduction of unknown forces into the treatment of disease meant that physicians untrained in the basic sciences on which a comprehension of these forces depends must begin anew their period of infancy and education, or yield their patients and their livelihood to those better informed. So far as electrotherapy is concerned, physicians have felt, no doubt with reason, that they must be shown. Whether this fortunate scientific skepticism was founded on a scientific frame of mind, or was merely an obstinate resistance to what was apparently an incomprehensible phase of medical treatment, is a matter for conjecture. In any event, the inspired pioneers of electrotherapy have had little patience with opposition, no doubt feeling that it was not based on comprehensive understanding of the things which to them seemed as simple as the child's alphabet. Let us, with editorial judgment, take the middle ground. No doubt the position of the medical profession regarding physical therapy has been unreasoning and blind; but just as certainly the enthusiasms of the pioneers were a beautiful manifestation of the credulous will-to-believe. Science demands controlled observations; it requires due precautions against the will-to-believe, definite allowance for the *vis medicatrix naturæ*, and simple admission that there is much that we do not know. The repetition of these aphorisms may sound as infantile as the squeaky "mamma" of the Christmas doll; but, alas, how necessary the repetition seems to be! When the allowances are all made, it seems that more must be granted at this time to those who opposed than to those who proposed, in the field of electro-therapy.

With the passing of time, the pioneers began to adapt themselves for the most part to the knowledge that medicine began to acquire from the fundamental sciences. The discoveries in chemistry, in physics, in biology, in physiology and in pathology began to make themselves felt in the physical therapeutic field. If one scans the reports made through the passing years, the names of masters of these related fields will be found in the records. Always apparent is the intent to eliminate the unscientific, to determine the actual physical basis of apparatus and of methods, to detect physiologic and pathologic changes such as may have occurred.

THE TEACHERS OF PHYSICAL THERAPY

Education in physical therapy to-day may be had through the available literature, represented by advertisements, pamphlets, articles in periodicals and text-books; through courses in physical therapy given by well-established schools and hospitals, by the paid representatives of manufacturing concerns, and by impromptu teachers with no credentials other than a profound belief in their own erudition; through the suave representations of detail men who know well how to befuddle the brain of the busy practitioner with a nomenclature fit for nothing so much as the construction of cross-word puzzles. Indeed, like all the literature of medicine, of art, of science, of religion and even of literature itself to-day, that of physical therapy may be divided into two main groups—the commercial literature and the literature of science. The groups infringe on one another to the extent that the literature of commerce is scientific and that the literature of science is commercial. Even a moron might follow easily the path of commerce or of science; but the unenlightened physician who wishes to tread the devious path between will need a guide to prevent him from straying into blind alleys and treacherous by-paths, and, indeed, from losing his way altogether.

At the meeting of the Modern Language Association held in Chicago recently, William McFee suggested that the American literature of the future would perhaps be the literature of commerce rather than the literature of science and of art. Since commercial organizations demand and pay for the best available literary talent, the magazine of the future may well consist of a central section of advertising written by masters in the literary field, surrounded by the rather dull pages of fiction produced by apprentices in the trade. Of course, even under the present arrangement it is hard to tell where the fiction ends and where the advertising begins in many periodicals. The cautious purchaser never forgets that the aphorism "Whose bread I eat, his song I sing" represents the psychologic observation of centuries.

The literature of commerce is a literature of affirmation; search as one may through page on page of circular, bulletin or advertising pamphlet, the statement of negation is a rarity. The literature is inspirational, leading inevitably to the signature on the dotted line. Even the most stupid of readers must already have noted the application to the field of electrotherapy of the fundamental psychologic fact discovered perhaps by Messrs. Macfadden and Hearst and widely exploited in their periodicals. Most of the illustrations used in the folders on physical therapy, observant readers have pointed out, represent the application of physical therapeutic methods, not to unfortunate soldiers, coalminers and teamsters, but to beautiful damsels, apparently in the pink of health, who have unveiled quite excessive portions of their intimate anatomy for the local application of a one-square inch electrode or the application otherwise of the healing heat or invisible ray.

The literature of electrotherapeutics, as I have intimated, comes sometimes frankly with the mark of commerce stamped on its pages; sometimes camouflaged behind the name of a physician who obviously is in the employ of, or has most certainly been influenced by, the concern devoted to the sale of the particular device. Frequently it is nevertheless the earnest effort of a sincere scientist to record his honest observations for the good of his fellow-physicians and for the benefit of mankind. Actually, the field of physical therapy is not nearly so bestrewn with the flimsy invitations of verbose commercial barkers as was the field of drug therapy at its worst some twenty-five years ago. There are, and have been, in the electric manufacturing field producers who have seen that permanent business demanded soundness from the start. They have proceeded cautiously in the issuing of advertising matter. They have attempted to state the facts concerning their devices and left it to scientific observation by clinicians to provide the claims. On the other hand, some manufacturing concerns have champed impatiently at the delay in adoption of their devices by cautious members of the medical profession. These business men, not content with the scientific observations made in well-controlled laboratories and clinics, have gone afield for the provision of their material, or have purchased the full time of easily credulous and perhaps not too meticulously ethical observers to supply claims for their machinery. The statement is a broad one, but it will be supported in due time by documentary evidence.

An investigation of the curriculums of medical colleges indicates that but few are ready to give courses in this branch of medical treatment. A survey of the hospitals of our country finds few of them adequately equipped with physical therapeutic apparatus; many are supplied with obsolete and inefficient, perhaps sadly rusted and degenerated, types; still others, equipped in the heyday of some lax political appropriation, present whole edifices devoted to intricate apparatus, both good and bad, which lie idle because of the lack of competent men and women to manipulate them. In this situation the practitioner turns naturally to possible sources of information.

The physician is informed by one concern or another that he may secure the privilege of instruction from an expert who is endowed by the manufacturing concern which promotes him with nothing short of celestial wisdom. The courses are offered free or for nominal sums, but are nevertheless commercial courses. Try as it may, the manufacturing concern which endeavors to promote the sale of its devices by the direct teaching of the physician cannot separate its teacher from the charge of commercialism. That teacher may be honest, his intentions may be of the best, he may even attempt to lean backward to avoid the taint of commercialism; but, as the poet eulogized:

You may break, you may shatter the vase if you will,
But the scent of the roses [?] will hang round it still.

Contrast with the flaming promulgations of commerce the modest announcement of the course in physical therapy offered by a university. Here is no blatant shouting of unusual virtues; merely the statement that the course has been planned for licensed practitioners of medicine only, that it includes six weeks of daily clinical work together with suitable lectures, and that it is offered to provide a working knowledge of the subject. Here is no announcement that physical therapy will bring to the practitioner taking the course extraordinary and increasing fees; no statement that the use of these electrical devices will win for him such practice as is now secured by self-advertising cultists; no inducement on the grounds that the flashy apparatus, issuing dazzling sparks and quivering rays, will attract to his books the misguided morons who are unable to distinguish between sense and sensibility. Here is the contrast between science and charlatanism.

Unfortunately the text-books, like the science itself, are undergoing a process of development which makes difficult dependence on any one of them. The most conservative find it necessary to limit so greatly the field of electrotherapeutics, and even of light therapy apart from therapeutics, that the practitioner is likely to consider its study, and most cer-

tainly investment in apparatus, little worth while.
On the other hand, the enthusiastic outbursts in
volumes by accepted leaders in this field are a strain
on the credulity of the most mellow of minds. One
author considers that "one of the most effective
uses of electricity is the relief, and at times the
cure, of all degrees of descension of the uterus,
except possible complete procidentia." "It is
probable," he asserts, "that every puerperal woman
would be the better for a course of nongalvanic
rhythmic currents after cessation of the lochia."
He advises "cathode depigmentation" for the removal of freckles; electric ionization for the cure
of salpingitis, and, in fact, finds some use for electricity in every possible physical or mental condition
that afflicts the human body. Actually, he recommends the treatment of ectopic gestation by electro-
cution of the fetus before the fourth month, and
the use of more moderate currents afterward to
promote its absorption. He wisely suggests that
in the meantime the patient should be at absolute
rest in bed, with the constant attendance of a nurse.

And yet these statements of presumably scientific
writers on electric therapy are mild indeed compared with the lucubrations of the commercial
wielders of the pen who are inhibited by no scientific doubts whatever in their development of literature that will sell the goods. Speaking of the incandescent lamp, one of them says:

When you use a thermotherapeutic light, you invoke nature's strongest force, the most permanent therapeutic power.

Another statement says of diathermy:

No physician's office, no hospital or sanitarium is complete without some good physical therapy equipment—particularly a diathermy apparatus of the portable or semiportable type. Such a machine is a very decided requisite if modern methods of medicine and surgery are to be employed.

Just how much more requisite a "decided requisite" or a "very decided requisite" may be than something that is just "requisite" deponent sayeth not.

And finally, for it would be possible to multiply these examples interminably, hearken to this section on "Resuscitated Sunlight":

We are all familiar with the marvelous vitalizing, beautifying and regenerating power of Sunlight. We have seen the earth, brown and sear in early Springtime, quicken to life and beauty; the tiny buds burst their prison cells, and develop into flower and fruitage; the fetid odors of putrescence disappear—and all, under this magic influence of the sun's rays.

Yes, more; we have watched with keenest interest the red blood come into the veins, sparkle into the eye and vigor into the limb of the anemic and invalid, through the stimulating effects of the "Sun Bath." But somehow, we limit the Electric Light to its luminous qualities, forgetful that in it we have real "bottled sunshine" under our absolute control, ready for application when desired and with the widest range of adaptation.

As the physicist has learned, the Electric Light is identical with Sunlight; in fact, it is Sunlight resuscitated from the energy long stored in the lumps of coal used as fuel. This latent energy in the coal, liberated in the furnace and transformed in the dynamo, is flashed forth again in radiance from the electric arc, or incandescent filament, on its interrupted mission of service to the world. In other words, that subtle force—that potent silent process that tints the petals of the lilac and the lily, that scents the rose and the jasmine, that flavors the ripening fruit in the orchard—is one and the same of Nature's forces, whether at work in the flower garden, on the sands of the seashore, or in the Light Baths.

It is presumed that the gentleman who wrote this statement is now more gainfully employed selling lots in Florida.

The physician who is anxious to perfect himself in the fundamentals of physical therapy, or even in the practical use of the apparatus, is confronted by a troublesome situation. As has been intimated, the schools of medicine and the post-graduate schools offer but few courses, and those not continuously. Moreover, mushroom schools have sprung up here and there to offer such courses to any aspirant, be he chiropractor, osteopath, cosmetician, chiropodist, barber, farmhand or blacksmith. Who has defined the point at which the work of the physical therapy aide or technician ends or commences? The ignorant cultist, licensed by a too-complaisant state to practice some single system of diagnosis and treatment, finds his patients seldom inclined to inquire whether or not his fundamental training warrants the use of the potent electrical devices with which he may have equipped himself. Indeed, most often this course of study has embraced some hours with the detail man or demonstrator and a cursory study of the book of directions, if he happens to be able to read. Even the "Naturopath" equips himself with artificial sunlight against the day when the clouds obscure the sky, although information has not yet been received that he has secured artificial grass and bottled dew for his nightgown-clad hypochondriacs to walk in while the artificial sun may shine.

The medical practice acts of our individual States make strange allowances for all sorts of unusual encroachments on the practice of medicine. Legislators seem not yet to have realized that the ability to diagnose disease according to the facts of modern scientific medicine is, and legally should be, an absolute prerequisite to any sort of treatment. The nurse, the technician, the aide, or whatever high-sounding title may be conferred on a medical as-

sistant, gains confidence with time and soon wishes
to depart from the sheltering wing of the physician
whom she may assist, to establish herself in her self-
constituted profession of physical therapist.   In
several States the new laws regulating the practice
of cosmetology specifically exempt the other new
profession of electrology so far as concerns the
removal of superfluous hair, moles, warts or excrescences from the skin.   There is need for some
body, with all the power and authority of organized
medicine in its support, to set forth above everything else the dangers of the ignorant employment
of electrical devices.

CHAPTER IX

PSYCHOANALYSIS—A CULTIST MOVEMENT?

I

THE human mind is unfortunately so constituted that but few persons ever learn judgment; most align themselves promptly on one side or another of every thought or conception thrown into the field of conversation or controversy, and are then ready to offer up their life's blood if need be in defense of the views that they have adopted. The pendulum of thought is then never still but always toward one extreme or another, the pull upon it of the enthusiasts on either side being far greater than the pull at the central point, where the experience of the past would indicate it more properly belongs. A good Freudian, reading this analogy, will immediately find in the pendulum one symbol and in the central point another; and I will be immediately convicted of repressions and other major crimes in the Freudian category from which it is difficult even for so serious and careful a person as myself to escape.

The Freudian doctrines came upon the psychological scene in 1894, apparently after Sigmund

Freud of Vienna had spent a brief period of study with Janet, noted French psychiatrist. Whether for reasons of internationalism or perhaps because of simple jealousy the French scientist has never been quite able to forgive Freud the development of his new school of thought. One cannot call it psychology, for the psychologists have in general repudiated most of it. The practice is properly the practice of medicine but the invasion of the field by hordes of quacks has made its very name anathema to most reputable psychiatrists. The educators have found the subject most thrilling in its application to the routine dullness of the educator's ordinary life. Hence it is that the finest blossom of this tropical plant is its relationship to the care of the growing child and its use for delving into the mind of the sexually precocious adolescent. In any event, Janet claims this fragrant offshoot with one hand while he repulses it with the other in the following reminiscence of the Freudian visit:

At this time a foreign physician Dr. S. Freud came to Salpetriere and became much interested in these studies. He granted the truth of the facts and published some new observations of the same kind. In these publications he changed first of all the terms that I was using: what I had called psychological analysis he called psychoanalysis; what I had called psychological system . . . he called a complex. He considered a repression what I considered a restriction of consciousness; what I referred

to as a psychological dissociation, or as a moral
fumigation, he baptized with the name cathar-
sis. But above all he transformed a clinical
observation and a therapeutic treatment with a
definite and limited field of use, into an enor-
mous system of medical philosophy—the philosophy of Pansexuality.

Janet is not, moreover, the only critic of the
Freudian school who insists that Freud derives
largely from other schools of thought. The difficulty of tracing the derivations lies in the fact that
the Freudian school has developed an entire nomenclature to facilitate converse among the elect, much
as a group of recalcitrant youngsters adopts a sort
of hog-Latin to keep its transactions away from the
juvenile bourgeoisie. Some of the critics refer to
the doctrine of purification of the emotions evolved
by Aristotle. Others mention Mesmer and his healing by hypnosis. Many insist that the entire system
is simply an elaborate ritual for conveying suggestion without the laying on of hands. Perhaps the
associated technique is sufficient to make the laying
on of hands an extremely elementary process by
comparison.

2

The basic conception of Freudianism is the comprehension of the "unconscious." This is the portion of the mind which is not directly responsible

for carrying on the functions of human existence that are simple processes in addition—and yet by the Freudian conception the unconscious enters into every human activity. It seems indeed to be the powerful minister behind the throne who insidiously guides the monarch—the conscious mind—into any plan that it desires. The unconscious has been described as a "magic cave where, by psychoanalysis, one can discover anything one puts into it." The most carefully reasoned presentation of the Freudian unconscious in brief form must be credited to Morton Prince. He considers that it embraces only mental processes that have been repressed from or kept out of consciousness because intolerable by reason of their unmoral, unsocialistic, and other characteristics; that for the most part never have entered awareness and therefore have been unconsciously and automatically kept apart; that are essentially of infantile origin and nature, the splitting of the mind into conscious and unconscious regions having taken place in the earliest part of childhood, probably in the first year; that involve the crude primitive instincts; that are predominantly sexual in character; and that, as they, necessarily like all processes, are dynamic, are sexual wishes. Morton Prince dismisses these views with the simple statement that they are not true, not confirmed by methods of research and, indeed, actually contradicted by scientific observations. Sachs, viewing the orgy of filth that arises from any one's unconscious when an adept Freudian disciple becomes active, blurts that "what Nature in her wisdom assigned to the unconscious had better remain there." Yet the Freudians would have it that this "Unconscious" is the dominating factor in our lives and that not only mental disturbances but phenomena such as pain, convulsive seizures, nervous coughs, spells, states of anxiety, images of compulsion, hallucinations and illusions are simply the symbols by which this Unconscious reveals itself to the outer world.

Any one will grant that the human being avoids disagreeable experiences and prefers not to think about them. It may be admitted that the eye constantly sees, the ear hears, the hands feel and the nose smells without positive recording of the impressions concerned. No doubt, the infant before arriving at the age of memory or reason is automatically receiving certain impressions. Then, too, all of us inherit forms of body structure, perhaps particularly brain structure, which may be concerned in our methods of thought and action. Certainly the will to survive, the desire to reproduce, the wish to satiate hunger, are fundamental in man as in the lower animals. But the Freudians would have it that these things are the impelling motives and that they seethe about in this Unconscious ever ready to burst forth against their owner's will. To prevent their eruption their owner represses them or holds them down consciously and this conflict between conscious and unconscious is the basis of all sorts of nervous and physical disorders, which are relieved, as we shall hear later, by psychoanalysis.

The German internist Bümke hesitates to accept such a complicated explanation of the situation. He recognizes that there is a crossing of several motives in the case of most human convictions and actions, and that the real reason for a certain act is not always that which appears most logical but very often one based largely on emotions. "Numerous contradictions arise in the life of a person," he says, "and it is these contradictions that we often discover in a disguised form in many neurotic individuals. Whoever is acquainted with the rationality of such an occurrence will, without the aid of psychoanalysis, have no difficulty in bringing out the truth and rid the patient from his troublesome complexes."

As has already been emphasized the sexual factor looms largest in the Freudian doctrines. All Freudians are agreed on the place of the unconscious but they are not so uniform in their acceptance of the place of sex as the prime factor in the unconscious. Indeed, they resort to strange evasions when the critics attempt to fix them definitely on this point. What was formerly understood by love— namely sexual love—has been gradually expanded into a new and much broader usage of that term. The Freudian "libido" embraces far more than could as notable a lover as Brigham Young. In the most recent enunciation of Freud himself "we call by that name the energy (regarded as a quantitative magnitude, though not at present actually measurable) of those instincts which have to do with all that may be comprised under the world 'love.' The nucleus of what we mean by love naturally consists (and this is what is commonly called love—and what the poets sing of) in sexual love with sexual union as its aim. But we do not separate from this—what in any case has a share in the name love—on the one hand self-love, and on the other love for parents and children, friendship and love for humanity in general and also devotion to concrete objects and to abstract ideas. Our justification lies in the fact that psychoanalytic research has taught us that all these tendencies are an expression of the same instinctive activities; in relations between the sexes these instincts force their way toward sexual union, but in other circumstances they are diverted from this aim or are prevented from reaching it through always preserving enough of their original nature to keep their identity recognizable (as in such features as the longing for proximity, and self-sacrifice). . . . Psychoanalysis then gives these love instincts the name of sexual instincts, *a posteriori,* and by reason of their origin."

The technique of psychoanalysis both as a method of diagnosis and of cure seems to be essentially simple, yet the great prophet himself insists that one cannot become a good psychoanalyst without a visit to the fountain head in Vienna, that one cannot be

a psychoanalyst until one has been himself submitted
completely to the complete process, and that the
fountain-head technique is the only technique. There
exist several tomes in which disciples have endeavored to describe the technique in detail. But
just as chiropractic split from or derived from osteopathy, so also have a dozen or more other schools
of psychoanalysis derived from the original school,
and new tricks of technique have originated with
them. In a recent promulgation one direct apostle
insists that the average time for an analysis is from
six to eight months with five or six sessions each
week. One ritual demands that the patient lie upon
a couch in a dimly darkened office. There she—and
the word falls naturally for it is usually a feminine
patient—begins her long autobiography and there
the psychoanalyst sits—we hope—listening and
stimulating ever more and more juicy revelations.

3

If there is ever a period in which the unconscious
is at its best, that time is when a person dreams.
Certainly his conscious cannot be dominating because
it is impossible when actually asleep to dream what
one wishes. Those who dream while awake have no
difficulty however in accomplishing in their fantasies
the things they desire. The Freudians have it that
the dream accomplishes what the unconscious desires—it is a wish-fulfillment. Obviously the ac-

tivities of the personnel involved in the dream are modified not only by all of the person's past experience, indeed even by his prenatal state, but also by all recent events and particularly by events of the day. The good psychoanalyst begins promptly to delve into the inner meanings of the dreams of his patients. It is at this point that the dirty work begins.

During the dreams the censor, that mythical controller of the complexes, is still active but not so wide awake, as when the person concerned is about his daily affairs. However, the censor continues to function sufficiently to cause the unconscious to adopt disguises for the persons and the ideas that are exploited in the dream. These symbols of things and persons have been organized to a certain extent but their possibilities are limited undoubtedly only by the limits of imagination of the psychoanalyst who is interpreting the dream. For instance, sex activity may be symbolized either by flying or falling, by going upstairs or by going downstairs, by riding, by fighting, by anything. The organs of sex are symbolized by hundreds, actually thousands of objects, usually of the most ordinary varieties of things occurring in daily life. In a dream analyzed by Jung, the patient dreamed of a certain number. "By adding in an ingenious way the figures for the year, month, and day of birth of the patient, of the patient's wife, his mistress, and his two children," says Dunlap, "the total gave the number, which is therefore the symbol of the patient's domestic triangle." Again and again these dream analyses fall into a *reductio ad absurdem*, but it remained for S. A. Tannenbaum, in the *Journal of Abnormal Psychology*, to investigate one of the dream analyses made by Freud himself, and to convict the great master of an apparent deliberate faking of a dream to prove a point.

It has been urged that psychoanalysis is a scientific method. Unfortunately no two psychoanalysts seem to agree in the interpretation of a dream. In one instance reported in the scientific literature two analysts differed as to an interpretation. The matter was referred to Freud and to Jung, and two additional interpretations were secured. A scientific method yields the same result every time. Actually, this variation of result and this continuous correction of the experiment to get a result that will fit the picture throws the method completely out of the scientific field. "When in interpreting a given phenomenon, as for example, to take the stock phenomenon, a dream," says Morton Prince, "we have to apply one or more of the various theoretical mechanisms, such as conflict, repression, displacement, compromise, disguisement (to avoid the hypothetical censor), inversion, transposition, regression, projection, introjection, transference, dramatization, condensation, sublimation, fixation, compensation, etc.—when we have to do more or less of all this in order to connect an antecedent experience logically with the dream or other phenomenon under investigation, it is obvious—at least so it appears to me—that the method falls far short of having that exactness which scientific procedure requires, and becomes a source of a large number of possible errors."

In the dream the complexes find a stage for their dramatizations. Using the scientific method the complexes have been classified. Such conceptions as the Edipus or "mother" complex (the turning of the sexual desire of the boy toward his mother) ; the Electra complex (desire of the daughter for her father) ; the various perversions of sex desire; narcissism; the inferiority and superiority complexes are the talk of the day among the intelligentsia, the artists, the Greenwich villagers, and the other insectia that thrive in a half-intoxicated condition in Batik hung studios where the lights are low and the tobacco smoke thick enough to cut with a knife. On the relative importance of these complexes the psychoanalysts have waged bitter civil warfare. From Freud have derived the schools of Jung, of Adler, and of a half-dozen other well-known disciples such as Stekel, Ferenczi, Ernest Jones, and Otto Rank abroad, and Jelliffe, Brill, White, Kempf, and others in this country.

4

After Carl Jung of Zurich had studied psycnoanalysis under Freud he evolved a different conception of the urge that drives mankind. Whereas the Freudian libido denoted sexual energy the Jung urge manifests other than sexual activities. Indeed, Jung conceives of progression which is a striving forward and regression which would make man go back to the irresponsibility of infantile and prenatal life. This regression, let it be understood, is essentially the Freudian Edipus complex. Moreover, Jung is primarily responsible for that delightful form of after-dinner amusement known as the word association test. In this method of determining the complexes, the patient receives a list of words and is instructed to respond to each with the first word that comes into his mind. The time necessary for each response is measured. A delay in the time of response and the unusual responses indicate that the person is concealing something because of a conflict. Among some of the other indicators of the presence of a complex are repetition of the stimulus word, response to a word previously given, naming some object in sight, rhyming to the word given, no response, or failure to reproduce the same response on repeating the experiment. Jung is also the formulator of the classification of mankind into "introverts" and "extroverts," conceptions which he first introduced in his "Psychology of the Unconscious" and which he has recently expanded into the scope of a new volume. The introvert withdraws himself from reality and lives in the realm of thought. The extrovert is gregarious and a man of action. Finally

Jung must be credited with having taken the new school of thought into high society. His disciples, particularly in Chicago, have given great concern to the public prints; he has lectured with great pecuniary emoluments; his nomenclature runs from the tongues of the four hundred more glibly than "two no-trump."

Alfred Adler, major prophet of another off-shoot of the great Viennese school, puts the main emphasis on the ego instincts instead of on the sex instincts. The dominating impulse in life is for power and the urge toward security. The desire for superiority is a compensation for a feeling of inferiority that may be based on an actual or a supposed defect of the body of the person concerned. Neurotic symptoms represent to him a protest against a constitutional inferiority or an inferior position in life. For example, hysterical outbreaks in women are frequently a protest against the supposed inferior position of women in general. As outlined by Hunter the Adlerian conception relates degeneracy, genius and neurosis in the following manner: The degenerate succumbs to his inferiority for his compensation is unsuccessful. The genius completely compensates for his inferiority by remolding himself or reality to suit his purpose. The neurotic compensates for his inferiority by a fantastic creation. He denies reality and compensates in daydreams or in behavior that does not adjust him properly to his environment. Such power as he achieves is secured through sickness by which he compels others to his wants.

The great work of Adler that has reached general acceptance has been his coöperation with pedagogic methods in Vienna. He conceives of a large majority of children as discouraged, which is of course merely another way of saying that they suffer with the inferiority complex. The discouraged child has this discouragement for one of three reasons: An organic defect, such as deafness, a club foot, a disturbed digestion, or some similar weakness; because it is spoiled due to parents having yielded to all of its minor demands, so that it has learned to lean constantly on others for its security; or because it is a hated child and conceives of all of the world as its enemies. Assuming that every child seeks some goal in life, for all of us constantly strive upwards, the discouraged child meeting an obstacle makes its escape by lying, stealing, or some other abnormal conduct. This psychology makes it a simple matter to excuse criminal actions of all kinds, since obviously responsibility for such actions must constantly be fixed on circumstance. The pedagogic method involves a retracing of the history of the child to the point at which its progress was blocked. It is then shown the reasons for its attempt to escape and it is pointed out that the heroic action in striving for the goal is taking the right path through the obstacle or over it, and not by evasion. This conception of Adler's is generally accepted as a major contribution to pedagogy, since it has done much to correct evil trends in childhood.

When this conception is applied to neuroses in women or to the criminal actions of adults, it begins to assume the possibilities of a dangerous cult, since it teaches the doctrine that the individual is never responsible for his actions. In its pursuit of the cause of the neurosis, it must perforce lean heavily upon sex causes which titillate the imagination and attract the neurotic. It is significant that Heinrich F. Wolf, one of the chief Adlerian disciples, has just issued a volume on "The Strategy of Masculine Seduction," in which the technique of the modern Casanova is thoroughly elucidated. To this volume Adler himself contributes an introduction with the sophistic argument that the value of such an analysis will be to make it possible for women to resist such antisocial conduct. The work will also have the advantage, he suggests, of removing obstructions to love interests, and thereby prevent neuroses and antisocial conduct. Adler also remarks naïvely that whenever he has lectured on human psychology and has permitted the audience to ask questions, 70 per cent of the questions were concerned with the technique and problems of love.

The whole conception of defense mechanisms, the building up of psychic compensations, the refuge in fantasy or heroic dreams of those who are inferior, the notion that one whose vision is defective compensates for the power by an acquired delicacy of touch or hearing, was fully expressed by the Irish bull, that it was a surprising thing that whenever a man had one leg that was shorter, the other was always longer.

Stekel, one of the most popular writers for the public on psychoanalysis, unquestionably derives all of his popularity from his facility as an author in this field. Possessed of a magnificent imagination, he is never at a loss for a suitable case to prove his points. Indeed, many Freudians have urged that he is not averse to using his creative art in developing suitable case material for such purposes.

Every one has heard of these major prophets of psychoanalysis. Few know about the vast number of disciples with slight modifications or individual idiosyncrasies to whom suitable space might be allotted. In our own country, Kempf has tried to get a physiologic basis for most of the neuroses and the mental disturbances, with a view to securing greater medical acceptance. His psychoanalytic practice is confusedly intermingled with much stress on the glands of internal secretion and on the autonomic nervous system.

5

Among the most fascinating applications of psychoanalysis has been the attempt to apply this method to a study of the minor mental incidents of daily life. The Freudians would have it that the traveling man who tells an obscene story in the smoking compartment of a Pullman car is merely resorting to a form of exhibitionism that takes the place of an actual display of his sexual proclivities. The person who makes a slip of the tongue or a slip of the pen does so because he is anxious to conceal his real mental attitude in the matter concerned. Forgetting, for instance, it is alleged, may sometimes be due to repression of something which one is anxious to forget, and probably in the majority of instances a sexual wish. On the other hand, it has been urged by psychologists who have given much attention to the matter that persons frequently fail to remember simply because of a natural condition of disinterest, and perhaps still more often because their minds are fixed on matters which interest them a great deal more. Indeed, Morton Prince asserts that the whole problem of remembering and forgetting is subordinate to the fundamental problem of why we remember at all. Such daily incidents of life as repeated washing of the hands, the Freudians assert, are due to some occurrence, perhaps in infantile life, in which the hands were concerned in a sexual catastrophe. Actually a good Freudian, if there is such an animal in the opposite sense of the word, seems to be able to find some obscene cause for practically any action on which a person may fix his attention, or about which he prefers not to speak. On the other hand, the majority of more careful thinkers are inclined to believe that sometimes we forget because we simply "do not give a damn."

I have heard Adler say, I have read in the writings of Freud, and of others in this particular field, that every action of human kind, individual or social, may be explained by the psychoanalytic technique. The absolute apotheosis of the cult of psychoanalysis is perhaps best expressed by Trigant Burow of Johns Hopkins University in his recent screed on this topic. He is certain that psychoanalysis will explain both religious hysteria and war, and he continues:

> Our frenzied greeds, our national competition and usurpations rest upon definitely compulsive reactions within the national consciousness. Our market inflations and our financial depressions are but the fluctuating mental states that represent the manic and depressive phases of an unstable social cyclothymia.
>
> The superficial and naïve explanations popularly assigned as the real occasion for these manifestations—such, for example, as the alleged necessities of territorial expansion, international commercial competition, the urgency of tariff readjustment, race prejudice, nationalism, our economic franchise, the rights of the minority, etc.—all these manifest symptoms are but the unconscious rationalizations well calculated to repress from the social consciousness the real underlying occasions of our national neuroses. What is called capitalism,

Nordic superiority, bolshevism, fascism, class consciousness, one hundred per cent patriotism, industrial democracy, our fluctuating ratios of monetary exchange—all these and a thousand more are but mental states which, instead of being greeted by us as substitutive manifestations calling for definite analysis and adjustment, are universally accepted as bona fide expressions and their latent meaning remains completely unchallenged in its psycho-social implications.

The criticisms that have been leveled against the development of psychoanalysis as a department of medicine or as a healing cult have varied from the simple assertion of Joseph Collins that the medical profession by and large, the world over, repudiates Freud, his theory of neuroses and his system of therapy to the terrific indictment of Frederic Peterson that psychoanalysis is a species of voodoo religion characterized by obscene rites and human sacrifices. When the Freudian conception was first launched upon the intelligentsia it became the plaything of artists, litterateurs and critics. It succeeded in dominating the writing of May Sinclair and in devastating such merit as existed in the work of D. H. Lawrence and J. D. Beresford. In this country a host of callow novelists, including perhaps Evelyn Scott, Ben Hecht and the early Sherwood Anderson were enabled to make intricate introspective analyses of their own sexual misgivings. The contrast between the work of these writers and the careful analytic studies of Theodore Dreiser is apparent to any critical reader. Even the literary intelligentsia, however, are beginning to line up with the psychologists and the physicians in their hesitancy to accept absolute Freudian domination. This repudiation seems to have resulted in the establishment of the practice of psychoanalysis by amateurish performers primarily perhaps for their personal excitement, but secondarily for commercial gain. The invasion of the field by such pseudo-scientific writers as André Tridon, Harvey O'Higgins and William Walsh is evidence of the opportunity afforded for exploiting such literary tripe. Unfortunately some physicians have also lent themselves to similar exploitation.

6

The practice of psychoanalysis for the healing of disease is the point at which it invades the medical field primarily. Its use in the treatment of disease has been a part of medical practice since the beginning of time. The confessional of the Catholic church, relieving thousands of disturbed minds, as well as every method of faith healing that has ever existed, including Christian Science, Couéism, autosuggestion, amulets, charms, incantations, chiropractic, and the laying on of hands in general, can report hundreds of cures of persons who are not actually sick. It is, however, an entirely different process to apply such methods simply and directly for healing of neuroses with a full knowledge of the reason for the application and with a full knowledge of any organic defects that may exist in the person concerned, and to use all of the paraphernalia of the charlatan to attract ladies of leisure and unfortunate victims of sexual aberrations into a method of treatment requiring months of time and tremendous financial outlays.

Worst of all, the majority of good psychiatrists are convinced that the orthodox method of psychoanalysis as practiced by the out-and-outers in this field is distinctly wrong in principle and meretricious in practice; that it degrades the personality; produces harmful results and is in general indefensible. "One need not be a physician," says a competent authority, "to realize that an infant is suffering from constipation, nor does it require considerable experience in life to know that nervous women during a reception will occasionally put their fingers in their pocketbooks. The infant does not do this because it derives pleasurable satisfaction, nor does the nervous lady signify a sexual relationship by her act."

Men of long experience in the psychiatric field are able to produce numerous instances in which the psychoanalytic technique has been the prime occasion for a severe disturbance of mentality by turning a sexual interest into a sexual aberration. The careful physician is perhaps even more likely to be wary of a part of the Freudian technique, because apparently the only way the patient has of ridding himself of some of his most difficult complexes is to transfer them to the doctor.

The invasion of the field by psychoanalytic amateurs has finally resulted in setting up defensive reactions among the psychoanalytic medical practitioners. In Vienna the physicians' group demanded that one of the non-medical psychoanalysts discontinue his practice, although he was certified by the great Freud himself, and insisted that psychoanalysts who are not physicians have not the right to treat patients for disease. A federal ministry of public administration, as the highest authority, has been called on to consider an opinion delivered by the leading psychiatrist of Vienna to the effect that only physicians should treat patients suffering from mental disturbances. In their defense, the lay psychoanalysts set up the fact that in America psychoanalysis is not regarded as a branch of medicine, but is considered to be primarily in the field of pedagogics and spiritual guidance.

Notwithstanding this defense, the New York Psychoanalytic Society was compelled recently to adopt resolutions urging that the practice of psychoanalysis in the treating of mental disease be restricted to physicians and that even the psychoanalytic instruction of specialists engaged in anthropology, theology, law, pedagogy and social service be limited to the use of this training for the

interpretation of problems in the special fields concerned. Furthermore, these medical psychoanalysts
demand that the instruction be limited to those having at least the Bachelor of Arts degree, and above
all, unequivocal evidence of good moral character.

7

The Freudian school will not recognize the status
of any one in psychoanalysis unless he has himself
been through the procedure with Freud or his immediate lieutenant. The great apostle is himself the
founder of a school of which he is the despotic head.
It is asserted, as it has been asserted by many charlatans in other fields, that this is to protect the
method against quackery. On the other hand, a
scientific method is able to stand any type of study
or investigation. The psychoanalysts insist, as do
all cultists, on an "all or nothing" policy. When
criticized, they seek escape by evasion, yet they
urge that in every normal person sexual perversion
is latent, and they attempt to classify as erotogenic
every portion of the body that may in some manner
be involved in sexual pleasure. The use of sym-
bolism has been exaggerated to a point beyond
reason.

The great contribution of Sigmund Freud, as admitted by all of the critics, has been to attract
greater attention to the processes of the human

mind, to stimulate the acceptance of the mind as such in its relation to disturbances of personality; in other words, to recognize that the study of objective changes in the human body is not sufficient to account for mental aberrations. The psychology of everyday life, the views regarding the dualism of the human mind, and its fundamental modifications have been a tremendous stimulus to psychology and to psychiatry. They have modified pedagogics and have created the new profession of behaviorist.

The position of Freud in the history of psychology is secure, but it is not the position that has been assigned to him either by his friends or his enemies. Psychoanalysis cannot be said to-day to be in any sense of the word an established science—the time may come when it will be recognized as a significant portion of the science of the human mind.

CHAPTER X

ETHICS—MEDICAL AND OTHERWISE

THE physician, if he is the graduate of a reputable medical school, has perhaps been told again and again, by preceptors and teachers, that his is a profession of service. No doubt, the example of sacrifices observed in clinic, dispensary and outpatient departments have impressed this conception upon him even more. With his diploma, he receives an address on high aims and service and a copy of the "Principles of Medical Ethics" of the American Medical Association. Possibly he lays aside the little book to read after the celebrations and examinations associated with this period in his career have ended. Then he embarks on his interneship and, following that, enters medical practice. But he is hardly likely to consult the booklet of ethics again unless invited to speak on the subject before some organization, or until some occasion arises in which he believes his rights may have been transgressed. Then he sends for a new copy, only to find in all probability that the things he thought were there are not really there at all.

The average man believes that medical ethics were developed primarily for the physician, and with but little regard for the interest of the patient. He believes that the physician is compelled either by this system or by some legal requirement to come to every patient every time he is called.

The physician believes frequently that medical ethics demand that other physicians treat him at any time and to any amount without exacting a fee, and not infrequently that physicians give gratuitous service also to all members of his immediate family and the families of his more distant relations.

He is certain that the principles prevent another physician from "stealing" his patients, and he is not infrequently of the opinion that the principles of ethics were formulated primarily for the protection of the rights of the individual physician rather than for the rights of the group.

In other words, the physician is first and foremost a human being with all of the failings of human beings in other businesses and in other professions. He is likely, if he is that kind of a man, to think first of "number one." He may, if he has the instincts of a miser, put receipts above service. He may, if he is naturally quarrelsome and antagonistic, be constantly at outs with his colleagues and his patients. Yet, if he has obtained a reputation for master ability in diagnosis, in surgical technique, or in medical treatment, he may continue to have a tremendous practice and to maintain this practice against constant opposition.

In medicine, as in all other professions and trades,

results count. Fortunately, the men who are great in medicine are also likely to be great in heart, great in mind and great in spirit; but there are exceptions, and physicians know of them probably oftener and better than do the public. After all, the greatest prize that a physician can secure is the esteem of his fellow-craftsmen, not the easily procurable flattery of the credulous public.

The public seems to believe there is no way of telling a good physician, an ethical one, or a scientific one from an unethical or an ignorant one. In many instances, public judgment is based on the kind of car he drives, the church he attends, the social position of his wife, his whiskers, or the protuberance of his abdomen. Frequently, a 48-inch waist measure is taken as the equivalent of a 48-caliber brain. A man may be a good Elk, a first-rate Shriner, an excellent grand sachem of the Red Men, own his own home and be considered a remarkable doctor, and still not be able to tell whether a sinking pain in the pit of the abdomen is due to an inflamed gall-bladder or a gastric ulcer.

The principles of ethics now official in the American Medical Association are a gradual evolution of a series worked over and developed through many years. It is significant that the work emphasizes, first of all, the duties of the physician to his patient. These duties include service as an ideal, patience and delicacy as highly desirable qualifications, and full assumption of responsibility once a case has been undertaken. The principles of ethics emphasize that a physician is free to choose whom he will serve, but point out that he should respond to any request for assistance in emergencies or whenever temperate public opinion expects the service. Many a great merchant made his success on the same factors.

The second chapter is concerned with the duties of physicians to each other. The physician is told that he must be an honorable man and a gentleman, that he must conform to a high standard of morals and uphold the dignity of his profession.

Then comes the question of advertising. The solicitation of patients is unprofessional. The section dealing with this question is explicit, covering every possibility and leaving little doubt as to interpretation. But when all is said, the conclusion is actually that a man ought to conform to the customs of the community in which he lives. If it has been the custom to publish a business card in the country newspaper, the physician may do so; on the other hand, if this is not the custom, he may not do so.

The principles of ethics protect the individual physician against the commercial group by stating that no group of physicians, organized, as a corporation, may do any type of advertising that is not permitted to the individual. The difference in point of view here emphasized between medical ethics and those of business is clearly apparent.

Medicine has for years depended for its success on the personal relationship between physician and patient. The great leaders know that the maintenance of this personal relationship is essential. Hence, every phase of the principles of ethics is planned to protect the rights of individual physicians against any group of physicians with the commercial ideal primarily in mind.

It has been said that John Wanamaker and Marshall Field owed their successes to the idea that the customer is always right. In other words, the purchaser must be pleased, and he must be protected not only from the deceits of salesmanship but against his own folly. This, after all, is the type of personal relationship which must exist between the physician and his patient. A pleased patient, as the principles of ethics repeatedly state, is the best type of medical advertisement. Just as the old law of *caveat emptor* no longer prevails in modern business, so also do the principles of medical ethics proclaim, "It is unprofessional to promise radical cures; to boast of cures and secret methods of treatment or remedies; to exhibit certificates of skill or of success in the treatment of disease; or to employ any methods to gain the attention of the public for the purpose of obtaining patients."

The ethical physician will not prescribe or dispense secret medicines or other secret remedial agents. The analogy of this part of the medical code to the best type of modern business is perhaps the statement in the advertising of clothing of the percentage of wool or cotton which make its content. It is similar to the clear statement on fabricated silks that they are not actually silks.

The principles of ethics were set forth not as a threat but as an inspiration. Just as there are merchants who by their nature rejoice in the shrewd deception of the ignorant customer, just as there are egoists in the control of manufacturing industries who do not hesitate to place their personal wishes above the good of all, so also there are in medicine physicians who feel that their judgment in the matter of prescribing remedies is better than that of the Council on Pharmacy and Chemistry, appointed by the American Medical Association to establish what is sound and reliable in new remedies.

The fault is not in the principles of ethics; it is in the character of the men who have failed to be inspired by the ideals and the high principles of their leaders. One might indeed quote Shakespeare when Cassius is made to say, "The fault, dear Brutus, is not in our stars but in ourselves."

A patient lay seriously ill, his physician gave a sad prognosis and, after giving somewhat explicit directions as to his conduct, asked, "Now, is there anything else that I can get for you?" "Yes," said the patient weakly, "another doctor."

From time to time, the official representatives of American medicine have debated the question of consultation, bearing in mind that the interest of the patient is paramount.

Section one of this portion of the principles does not equivocate. "In serious illness, especially in doubtful or difficult conditions, the physician should request consultations." And it continues, "In every consultation, the benefit to be derived by the patient is of first importance. Time and again physicians argue the question as to consultation with irregular practitioners, or those devoted to the tenets of some sectarian practice or cultist system." The principles of ethics are not specific on this point, but there is a section devoted to the honor of the profession, which says: "A physician should not base his practice on an exclusive dogma or sectarian system, for 'sects' are implacable despots; to accept their thraldom is to take away all liberty from one's action and thought."

There are many physicians who refuse to recognize cultist practice, even to the extent of giving aid to a patient while the patient is still under the care or control of such a practitioner.

There are others who do not hesitate to come in and give advice to patients who may be under such care.

Above all, the physician must consider the good of the patient.

There are physicians who are careful to inquire of the patient as to whether or not he has seen a previous consultant and as to the opinions of the ones first consulted; there are others who are not too meticulous in determining this point. Indeed, a sagacious physician will know promptly from the information possessed by the patient whether or not he has been informed elsewhere concerning his condition. One is almost prompted to suggest that in these instances the wise physician will bear in mind the motto *"caveat vendor,"* just as the merchant must apply the same motto to the type of customer who shops too insistently and whose bills are likely to remain unpaid.

The principles of ethics recognize the fact that the medical diagnosis is usually paid for insufficiently in comparison with the reward of surgical technique. "The patient should be made to realize," say the principles of ethics, "that a proper fee should be paid the family physician for the service he renders in determining the surgical or medical treatment suited to the condition, and in advising concerning those best qualified to render any special service that may be required by the patient."

The third phase of the principles of ethics is again a recognition of the duty of the physician to the public. He is asked to remember that he is a citizen and to aid in enforcing laws and in giving advice concerning public health. During an epidemic, he must continue his labors for the alleviation of the suffering, without regard to the risk of his own health or life or to financial return. He is asked to warn the public against the devices practiced and the false pretensions made by charlatans, and he is told finally that these principles do not cover all of the obligations which he may have, but are wholly a guide which will supplement the ordinary conduct of a gentleman and the practice of the Golden Rule. The last sentence reads, "Finally, these principles are primarily for the good of the public, and their enforcement should be conducted in such a manner as shall deserve and receive the endorsement of the community."

Fellowship in the American Medical Association is contingent on the possession of this membership.

The Association maintains a Judicial Council which carefully considers complaints brought against any of the fellows or members for infractions of any of the principles of ethics.

But the number of complaints brought and the number of physicians expelled from fellowship or membership each year is surprisingly small!

CHAPTER XI

THE PHYSICIAN OF THE FUTURE

I

THE practice of medicine in our fair land is giving pause to the professional sociologists and economists and to the amateur medical philosophers. More and more the columns of our medical periodicals and the pages of our weekly publications devoted to thought (in italics) are concerned with the manner in which the progress of medical science is to be made available to the average man (in quotes). Perhaps never before in the history of medical affairs has there been such a profuse viewing with alarm and as much heated consideration of the topic "whither are we drifting." To this shrill soprano chorus of anxiety I interject a deep bass note of "Sailor, beware," for many brave ships are lost in the sea of prophecy and the old ocean rolls on in sullen scorn.

In the last century the knowledge of scientific medicine has advanced more than in the previous two thousand years. In the same period of time the ability of men to reason and to think has certainly not advanced by five per cent. and it is a question if it has advanced at all. Certainly the fundamental observations of the ancient philosophers as to ways of life have been little improved either as to content or form by the enunciations of the present. The pre-Christian Hippocrates, or the group of men now credited with having prepared the texts to which his name is given, did not lack in the ability to observe the manifestations of disease and was weak in interpretation of those manifestations only to the extent of lack of knowledge of certain facts of anatomy, physiology and pathology which have been the achievement of the intervening centuries. Those physicians were dependent, however, almost wholly on the five natural senses, whereas the medico of to-day has available all of the prolongations of those senses made possible by the X-ray, the electrocardiograph, the audiometer, the stethoscope, the microscope, the cystoscope, and thousands of similar devices. Moreover, the bedside practitioner is able to take from his patient not only the fluids excreted by the simple processes of nature but to remove by needle, tube, or other device any secretion or excretion that may be expectorated, eliminated, ejaculated or otherwise extricated from the system. These he need not examine for himself, for their study constitutes one of the most intricate of the medical specialties. He turns them over to a laboratory technician who, in time, makes available to him information of the utmost importance in determining the extents of the ravages of the patient's malady. Indeed, every one now recognizes that the field of medical knowledge is far too great for any one physician to be able to practice with equal competence all of its specialties and branches. Even the yokel who trusts in times of minor ailments to the tender mercies of chiropractor, Christian Scientist, or other faith healer, seeks out what he believes to be the most competent of medical specialists when disease threatens his organs of procreation.

The medicine of to-day is the outgrowth of the medicine of the past. Then a practitioner of compelling personality, wise in the ways of men, learned by observation, profound with knowledge accumulated slightly from books but far more from precept and case history and example, wrought the healing of disease by a knowledge of the value of food and of rest, by the use of a few simple remedies whose actions were known and of hundreds of remedies with no actions whatever. He relied most of all, as do all of the quacks and the cultists of to-day, on the *vis medicatrix naturæ,* the natural tendency of the body to get well anyway and on the fact that many common ailments seem to be self-limited. Medical science did advance, however, and with it hygiene and sanitation. Otherwise the life expectancy would still be at 35 where it was a hundred years ago instead of around 55 where it hovers ready to advance still further to-day. This increase of life expectancy came about through our knowledge of infectious disease and the control of infant mortality.

The difficulty with medical conditions to-day has been excellently expressed by George E. Vincent of the Rockefeller Foundation, who views not with alarm but with smiling cynicism. In an address delivered at the annual meeting of the Medical Society of the State of New York and in several pronouncements issued subsequently President Vincent has said that the medical profession does not function adequately in its delivering of the knowledge that is available. More than three-fourths of our population, he asserted, are treated by general practitioners who have limited technical appliances, little or no specialization of skill, and slight relation to medical services organized in hospitals, dispensaries and clinics. The rich, constituting five per cent. of our population, receive the best skill of well equipped specialists, and the poor, constituting fifteen per cent., receive similar skill through organized institutional practice. He charges also neglect of the psychic side of medicine, failure to educate the public, narrowly conceived professional policies, and great shortcomings in the knowledge, skill and integrity of a considerable number of our physicians. General practice is doomed, he prophesies, unless the general practitioner will submit to a measure of organization and team play in the coöperative use of laboratories and other resources, unless he will meet the demand for spreading costs of sickness over large groups through readjusted forms of compensation, and unless he will become more and more a practitioner of preventive medicine.

The change of emphasis from cure to prevention has caught the doctors napping. The average physician is ill prepared to make the periodic health examination and to give the advice about personal hygiene which the new régime demands; he has been trained to look for disease rather than for health. . . . Some time physicians will receive annual retainers to keep their clients in good running order. But before this system can be efficient, medical schools will have to turn out physicians who have been taught to do this special kind of work. . . . The aim then is to permeate the medical school with the preventive idea and to modernize the medical profession as a whole."

Thus President Vincent, as to the practice of medicine and some of its aspects.

From the sociological angle the learned Dr. Vincent sees further difficulties. The centering of practitioners in the cities is creating a serious situation, removing the patient in the country from prompt if not from competent attention, and making it difficult to apply in his case particularly the resources of the hospital and the laboratory. In the cities the principle of insurance, industrial groups with full time paid physicians, sick benefit societies, and lodges attempt to provide organized medical care at a low cost. Medical societies fear state medicine in any form, worse than the pest. Yet sociologists, and particularly socialists, see in government control of medical practice, in such legislation as the Sheppard-

Towner Act, and in similar conceptions for the control of the ailments of child, horse and man, of parturition, dysentery, hog cholera, syphilis and ophthalmia neonatorum, the cure for all of the difficulties of carrying modern medicine to the people.

One may not quarrel with this diagnosis but may differ greatly in the matter of therapy. The situation is perhaps analogous to that of the physician and chiropractor called in consultation on the same patient. The medical profession asks a minimum standard of knowledge for all who propose to treat the sick, regardless of the method of treatment used. A chiropractor, with such knowledge, would never use the chiropractic method of treatment. One expects a sociologist of the attainments and repute of President Vincent to make a better diagnosis of the social ills of our democracy than might be made by any one of a thousand physicians. But when he elects to specify the form which medical diagnosis and treatment are to follow in the future he treads on foreign soil, where he requires expert medical guidance. The situation is much as if a physician, using all the armament of modern medical science, should actually find a spinal vertebra out of place and pressing on a nerve, as might occur, let us say, in one of a million cases of disease which a physician might see. In such an instance it is conceivable that the physician might elect to have a chiropractor use a chiropractic thrust for a sudden readjustment of the correct alinement. It is far more likely that he would call upon an orthopedic surgeon, whose knowledge of the relationships of bones, ligaments, nerves and muscles is probably better than that of a chiropractor, a naprapath, an osteopath and a sanatologist combined. In brief, the diagnosis and treatment of the ailment of our democracy in the matter of its medical care is a problem requiring consultation of sociologist with economist, psychologist, physician and politician. It is to the results of such a consultation that I now address myself.

2

Sir James Mackenzie, a leader of British medicine for many years, in a volume on "The Future of Medicine" emphasized the conviction that the general practitioner must continue to be the fundamental factor in medical practice. To him the patients come—or should come—with the earliest symptoms or signs of disease. He alone knows intimately the family of the patient, his environment, his economic status. The specialist sees only too often the diseased organ and not the diseased man. Mackenzie, beginning life as a general practitioner, achieved such note for his diagnostic acumen that he passed soon to the rank of consultant. His epoch marking contributions to knowledge of the heart gave him world-wide fame as a specialist in that field. But general practice was his delight and to that he returned in his declining years.

In "Pygmalion, or the Doctor of the Future," Dr. R. M. Wilson, a disciple of Mackenzie, draws a vivid, compelling picture of a physician whose relationships to his patients will be even more intimate than those that present-day leaders demand. Wilson sees him as a great humanist—almost a priest, in a new sense of the word—a man with the widest possible knowledge of human nature, and the deepest possible understanding of human motives. This is, of course, the mark left on medicine by the influence of the Freudian doctrines.

Such clinicians as Billings, Pusey, Haggard, Lambert and Phillips, all presidents of the American Medical Association, such medically trained organizers and analysts as Work, now secretary of the interior, and Wilbur, president of Stanford University, also presidents of the Association, have insisted again and again that, come what may, the intimate personal relationship of physician and patient is fundamental to sound medical practice and absolutely essential to proper relief of the patient's ills.

Nevertheless, one finds opposed to these clinical reports the assertions of Vincent that the general practitioner does not serve efficiently. "Only in university clinics, in well developed hospitals, dispensaries and pay clinics, in true group practice, in health centers," he says, "is there to be found genuinely organized medicine, i.e., the teamwork of skillful diagnosticians with well trained specialists backed by efficient laboratory, operating and treatment facilities." Granted that such organizations may be mechanizing medicine, eliminating the personal factor and the human relation he sees them as advancement: "The specialization and organization are accepted as unescapable consequences of social changes." And his final prophecy is again perhaps well within some of the definitions of state medicine that have been mentioned. "It looks as if society means to insist upon a more efficient organization of medical service for all groups of people, upon distribution of the costs of sickness over large numbers of families and individuals, and upon making prevention of disease a controlling purpose."

In support of the views of Vincent, comes now one Joseph Krimsky, practicing physician of New York City, who pleads with his colleagues of the middle class to enter a government controlled medical service. He recognizes the onslaughts made by public health practice and by free clinics. He fairly yearns for a salaried position for every physician. And he has a sweet, Debs-like, faith in political control. Thus Dr. Krimsky in *The Nation*:

> Why not make the community pay you for your services in decent salaries rather than try to take it out of a rapidly dwindling private clientele? Is it beneath your dignity to be officers and employees of the public? Some of you are timid about the influence of politics on such a plan. An organized medical profession aiming at scientific advancement and having

the public interests as its goal will always have the public backing against any sinister political influences.

Indeed, Dr. Krimsky has all the credulity of all the socialists in his blind acceptance of the statistics provided by the promoters of social reforming schemes. He even believes that income tax reports are accurate.

Of all the contributions to this symposium of opinions—for after all one deals here primarily with opinion and not with fact—that of Dr. James B. Herrick is expressed with most scientific reserve. It is based, moreover, on a long experience in general practice and as a consultant. He sees a practitioner who will continue to be a human being much as now, who will continue to work for gain, reputation, opportunity and power. He hesitates to say whether socialism will or will not prevail but hopes for freedom from too rigid state control because repugnant to "our ideas of the dignity of the profession." He believes medical leaders are blinded to the shortcomings of the old time general practitioner—that they are swayed by sentiment and he looks toward a "new clinician, the general practitioner of the future, who without loss of the intimate personal relation will embody more of the man of learning."

But it is unnecessary to rewrite or condense the words of Herrick.

The new practitioner must know more of fundamental sciences and their application in

medicine, and must be better able to correlate
and to interpret the findings of specialists,
laboratories and instruments of investigation.
He must be capable of diagnosing the vast majority of ailments that come to his attention,
competent to treat a large proportion of them.
But of just as much importance, he must recognize his own shortcomings, must know when to
call in the specialist and which man to call.

"Whether we like it or not," says Dr. Herrick,
"specialism is here and is bound to stay, if not permanently, at least for a long season." The growth
of medical knowledge has made it impossible for one
man to grasp all of it. It is granted that specialism
also is in a stage of evolution, and that already
leaders in medicine are seeking for plans which will
permit the public to know specialists who are really
qualified from the pretender and the poseur.

Many specialists are such in name only, a
name often self-assumed. Many are narrow.
Many, poorly prepared, lack broad experience
and proper graduate study. They are often
more concerned with technic than with diagnosis or indication for treatment. Some are
offensively commercial. But in the future one
type of clinician will be the well qualified specialist. He will not be confined by any means
to our large cities; he will not be narrow. He
will be readily available; a man as considerate
of his fellow practitioner's reputation and com-
fort as he is of the patient's pocketbook. On
him must lean heavily the practitioner, incom-

petent to treat certain diseases and trained to admit his incompetence. The operation on gall-bladder or prostate gland, the dietetic management of the poorly nourished infant, the expert handling of the neurasthenic, the proper use in certain cases of roentgen ray, radium and perilous drugs, the skilled manipulation of instruments of precision or the technic of applied bacteriology and chemistry—these may be outside the practitioner's field. He must call in the specialist or take the patient to him. This is easy to-day, so easy, in fact, that the patient often goes to the specialist over the head of the general practitioner, particularly when the illness seems acutely dangerous or chronically baffling. Telegraph, telephone, good roads, the automobile and the small town hospital make specialists easily and increasingly available. With the growing popularization of medical knowledge, the general practitioner must learn to recognize the need of or the desire for the specialist, or often be left out altogether.

The relation between specialist and general practitioner must be more cordial, intimate and coöperative than now; they must be not rivals but colleagues, mutually helpful. Let the profession come out frankly and place the general practitioner on a higher plane of self-respectability by taking him in as a partner of the specialist. If necessary, let there be an open—not secret—sharing of a reasonable fee, at least in many cases. This will remove the now strong temptation for the practitioner to do himself, because of the urge for money, what he is really unfitted to do. The result of this partnership will inure to the benefit of the patient, who in spite of some of our medicine-as-a-trade advocates, is the prime consideration. The moment we fail to keep the ideal of benefit to the patient before us, practice will degenerate and will be in essence dishonest.

3

The consultants then have spoken and it remains, according to the Principles of Medical Ethics, for some one, after summing up the observations to prescribe the cure, or at least to venture a prognosis. What the cure will be only the passing of the years to a time far beyond our period will reveal. About a prognosis I am not so hesitant for the disease is an old one from which other nations and professions have suffered and are suffering.

The physician of the future must be a being of much the same type as that now prevailing among us. He will have the same variety of virtues and failings as other men in his community. He is likely, if he is that kind of man, to think first of himself; he may, on the other hand, be one of those sweetly sentimental souls that permits himself and his family to suffer, while he attends to everybody's business but his own.

If he has the instincts of a miser or the acquisitiveness of a Shylock, he will put receipts above service. Neither medicine nor any other profession, not excluding all of the Freudian, behaviorist or other psychologists, has evolved any test of character that will admit to medical schools or to medical practice only men of undoubted integrity, idealism or charitableness.   Neither is there any certain method for determining that the attributes of a character or mentality that stamp the man on entrance into the study of medicine will persist through the terrific demands of the modern curriculum or the pitfalls and stresses of modern medical practice. Scientists hint vaguely about the scientific type of mind but they recognize it by its results and not by any series of standards applicable before those results have been achieved. Out of the five or six thousands of young men who embark each year on the study of medicine there are inevitably many who are unfitted by nature, by heredity, by every possible criterion to study or to practice medicine. They are qualified undoubtedly by ability to study, and by income. But once in the groove the side walls of pride, of discipline, of competition and of weak placidity tend to keep them there. And how many are willing to sacrifice the seven years of study and the thousands of dollars spent upon the education in yielding up their rights to practice when the course is completed? From such unadapted weak sisters the profession of medicine suffers as much or more than any other profession in our midst.

A poorly informed complacent public selects, its healers as it selects its barbers and milkmen. Social position, the type of car driven, the waist measure, the church affiliations, and membership in Elks, Masons, Red Men, Rotary or Kiwanis Club are the determining factors. Whether he be osteopath, chiropractor or disciple of Macfadden makes little difference to a public that thinks gastritis means gas on the stomach. The misfit physician, fitted into such a community, soon realizes that his patients are satisfied with as little as he cares to give them. A community will have physicians as good as it cares to demand.

The modern physician swims a difficult course between the rocks of laboratory technique and the insidious whirlpools of careless diagnosis and faith healing. A complete study of his patient demands a vast number of technical tests which are not perhaps necessary for a suitable diagnosis of the cause behind the patient's chief complaint. Such a complete study is a time-consuming, painstaking, costly process to which few patients are yet educated and for which few patients are willing to pay. Nor are all of the tests necessary in every instance. The idealistic sociologist sees a future in which all men will have the benefit of these studies, reduced in cost and in time consumed because of a Fordizing of their application. The consummation will never be realized nor is it devoutly to be wished. In such standardization of medical practice science falls by the wayside in the facility of routine; sufficient unto the day is the completion of the job. The individual becomes no longer a living man or woman but a blood specimen, a sputum, a stomach, or a prostate. Already in the great group clinics the vernacular begins to refer to him in this way. The patient quickly becomes a case.

The physician of the future must then continue to be much as to-day—a man dealing with men. The general practitioners will be needed more than ever for the care of the simple derangements of human function, the relief of symptoms perhaps easily borne but better relieved, and above all, for sifting the major disturbance from the minor complaint. In that sifting he calls upon the aid of laboratories and roentgenographers for his diagnosis and for surgical, dermatologic, ophthalmologic, or other special technical aid for treatment and control.

The majority of parturitions are without complication and require only watchful waiting. The enlightened general practitioner will know when the required technical manipulations have reached a point beyond his competence. Such attentions are not to be had at the clinics or in the pamphlets provided by a solicitous government through the Sheppard-Towner idea.

The periodic physical examination is a magnificent conception for the detection of the degenerative disease in its earliest stages. But the human being will not receive these in the clinical mill provided by a government, a philanthropy, an industry or a commercial corporation with hired physicians. He will receive these from a competent family physician. And the physician will be paid by an individual who is receiving sufficient compensation from his employment to bear the expense of the examination. True, in these times, many industries are attempting to provide the examinations with full time salaried physicians; true, the Life Extension Institute attempts the plan on a corporation basis; true, groups of physicians organized in a business manner engage to do the work at a considerable fee. But as long as there are human beings witless enough to be satisfied with such methods of medical practice and willing to take these things as they are provided, there will always be those who are ready to provide. We live, alas, in a democracy, and the medical Utopia, even Samuel Butler's "Erewhon," is still far, far away.

4

Possibly the application of medical practice has changed by the development of the hospitals. The advantages lie in the ability of one especially competent physician to see many more patients in a single place where all the armamentarium of medical technique is assembled. But the disadvantages lie in a still greater depersonalization of the patient as he was seen at home. And hospitalization, too, continues to be a more and more costly process. The

rich can afford it.   The poor are provided with
it through the increasing burden of state aid and the
accumulation of vast philanthropies.   The middle
class, existing in the kitchenette, must perforce have
the hospital when it falls ill for even the obscenity of
nocturnal employment of the quarters devoted primarily to eating, bridge and listening to the radio,
cannot tolerate pneumonia, ozena, rheumatism or
even any of the complaints whose names end with
"rhea."   To the hospital then the middle class must
go and it pays as it always has and always will pay
for being the middle class.   The physician of the
future will deal largely with this group.   From them
most of the physicians, who are themselves of the
middle class, will derive their incomes.   The long-
suffering middle class has been in the habit of having
a middle class service from middle class physicians
and there will be provided, no doubt, as there are
already being provided more middle class hospitals.
But even Dr. Vincent knows that there will not be
provided the medical service that is given to a Rockefeller and for which a Rockefeller pays.

5

Group practice, either that provided by salaried
physicians, employed by corporations of business
men, or by stock companies, or partnerships of physicians who are good business men, have failed in the
past, are founded and fail in the present and will

no doubt continue to fail in the future.   Business is business and medicine is medicine and never the twain shall meet.   Doctors continue to urge and to demand a study of business methods under the name of medical economics but a sincere application of what are known as true business methods is incompatible with the ideals of medicine and means certain medical failure.

The principles of ethics protect the individual physician against the commercial group by stating that a group of physicians, organized as a corporation, may not do advertising that is not permitted to the individual.   Medicine depends for its success on the personal relationship between physician and patient. The thought of the professional group protects this relationship.   The group depends for its scientific position on what the individual members of the profession think of it; when they think badly, the group is already beginning to die a lingering death.

True, there are exceptions to the rule.   The Mayo Clinic, the Battle Creek institution and perhaps a hundred other clinics manage to progress but in each instance some unusual personality or some extraordinary factor may be found to explain the exception.   For the mass of medical practice the plan is unavailable.   The clinics live by the grace of the general practitioners.   Without them there could be no clinics.

6

What then of state medicine? The system is unthinkable. It has never succeeded anywhere on a large or a small scale. State medicine might, indeed, provide a standardized diagnosis and treatment for a standardized citizen. If medicine were chiropractic, state medicine would be quite compatible with its practice. But it is the death of initiative, of humanity, of science. It attracts the type of mind that makes a four hundred dollar motor car. Until we become a nation of Robots with interlocking, replaceable and standardized parts, there will be little chance of such completely standardized doctors.

For years the medical profession has been considered a profession of humane service. The young man entering medicine represents an investment of six to eight years of time during which he not only sacrifices the money he spends in securing an education, but the money he might have earned and the income from both the sums; an amount calculated at from $12,000 to $15,000. In return for this he has been enabled to look forward to a leading position in the social organism, with the possibility that after several additional years of toil and striving he may be able to make a fair living. What if he is to look forward instead to a salaried position in a large organization in which he automatically follows a narrow routine? He is no longer a physician; he is

no longer treating human beings for the relief of
their ailments. He has become a tonsil mechanic,
an adjuster of adenoids, or an inspector of gonor-
rhea. The prospect is not one likely to appeal to
the type of man who now becomes a physician; it
would not attract even a chiropractor or a Christian
Science healer.

7

The evolution of modern medicine was a gradual
process until the great discovery by Pasteur of the
causative relationship of bacteria to disease. With
that discovery came a great impetus from which developed modern sanitation and hygiene with a prolongation of the average human life. There has
been, however, but little average prolongation of
life beyond the age of seventy, and there is not the
slightest scientific reason to believe that there ever
will be. The general extension of human existence
will undoubtedly bring new problems of overpopu-
lation and of economic adjustment in daily life. It
is unreasonable to believe that medicine will play
any great part in solving this question, unless it develops, as it may, some system of immunization
against conception. But even this will be used by
the intelligent and avoided or misused by the un-
intelligent.

Quackery, cultism and frauds of all types will
continue to take their toll among the ignorant who

are uninformed, and among the educated who know enough to be easily misled. The fertile mind of the quack avails itself of new plans as rapidly as scientific medicine develops new ideas for human benefit. It is inconceivable that the time will ever come when the percentage of persons misled by quackery will be greatly reduced, except to the extent that the coming generations are educated in the fundamental facts concerning the human body. But even here the prejudices of puritanism and prudery delay progress. The outlook for the prompt establishment of a medical Utopia seems pessimistic—and it is.

THE END